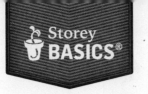

Storey
BASICS®

HERBS for CHILDREN'S HEALTH

How to Make and Use Gentle Herbal Remedies for Soothing Common Ailments

Rosemary Gladstar

Storey Publishing

*The mission of Storey Publishing is to serve our customers by
publishing practical information that encourages
personal independence in harmony with the environment.*

Edited by Nancy Ringer and Melinda A. Slaving
Series design by Alethea Morrison
Art direction by Michaela Jebb
Text production by Theresa Wiscovitch
Indexed by Nancy Wood

Cover illustration by © Meg Hunt
Interior illustrations by Alison Kolesar, 15; Beverly Duncan, 32, 55, 80, 84, 86;
  Brigita Fuhrmann, 43; Charles Joslin, 9, 51; Louise Riotte, 30; Sarah Brill, 20, 25,
  27, 37, 44, 46

This publication is intended to provide educational information for the reader on the
covered subject. It is not intended to take the place of personalized medical counseling,
diagnosis, and treatment from a trained health professional.

Storey Publishing
210 MASS MoCA Way
North Adams, MA 01247
www.storey.com

Printed in the United States by Versa Press
10 9 8   7   6

LIBRARY OF CONGRESS CATALOGING-IN-PUBLICATION DATA

Gladstar, Rosemary, author.
  Herbs for children's health / Rosemary Gladstar.
    p. ; cm. — (Storey basics)
  Herbs for children's health
  Includes bibliographical references and index.
  ISBN 978-1-61212-475-9 (pbk. : alk. paper)
  ISBN 978-1-61212-476-6 (ebook : alk. paper)
  I. Title. II. Title: Herbs for children's health.
  [DNLM: 1. Plants, Medicinal—Popular Works. 2. Child—Popular Works. 3.
  Phytotherapy—methods—Popular Works. QV 766]
  RJ53.H47
  615.3'21083—dc23
                    2014048736

CONTENTS

Preface v

CHAPTER ONE: **Herbal Medicine for Children** 1

CHAPTER TWO: **The Best Herbs for Children** 10

CHAPTER THREE: **Treating Common Childhood Ailments** 33

CHAPTER FOUR: **How to Make Herbal Remedies** 88

Recommended Reading 117

Resources 118

Index 120

To all of the earth's children, small and large, young and old.
May we steward the plants and the earth they grow upon
in such a way that they remain in sweet abundance for
future generations of plant lovers, so that when you walk
upon the land with your grandchild's hand
in yours, you can show them the
same sweet medicines of the earth.

As I was finishing the last pages of the first edition of this book, my young nieces Samantha (then age 10) and Lindsey (age 6) were coming over to spend a night with their "Aunt Rosie" so we could share a day of herbal delights. *"I've been planning for the last few days the things I wish to do with them,"* I wrote. *"There's so much that's green and beautiful and so many wonderful things to do with plants. We'll make my famous herbal face cream, make lip balms, and maybe do herbal steams and facials."* These young girls are fully grown now, and they both still have that deep love of the earth and its natural gifts that was nurtured in their childhood.

My granddaughter Lily is next in line to come to Grammy's "School of Herbal Healing." Lily, already eight years old, has grown up on an herb farm and knows her herbs quite well. Recently she invited her entire class on a field trip to her family farm, Zack Woods Herb Farm. Though her parents were there to help, it was Lily who took her fellow students on an herb walk, proudly pointing out the wild plants and the rows of neatly growing medicinal herbs. She had fun instructing her friends how to use them in salves, in teas, and as poultices, and judging by their enthusiasm and excitement, the kids were all interested.

We'll be taking Lily camping in a few days, and just like when her older cousins came to visit, I have planned an assortment of activities that are plant-related. We will make plant presses to press some of the common wildflowers and leaves for her first herbarium. I'll remind Lily why we don't pick some of the woodland plants growing around our campsite — either because they are rare, so we want to help protect them, or else because some plants, like poison oak, protect themselves with toxic oils that cause a painful rash to those who are foolish enough to grab them. We'll also make a special campers' flower essence to remind us of our trip together. And maybe on one of the warm summer evenings we'll stop to watch the fireflies and tell the stories that the trees are whispering to us. . . .

It is at times like these that I am reminded most of my own early encounters with plants. I am forever thankful for the lessons my grandmother taught me as a child in her gardens. Though I have gone on to study plants with great teachers and have traveled around the world to learn ever more about them, it is still those teachings that I learned at the feet of my grandmother that were planted the deepest and have stayed with me the longest. No matter how little you think you may know about the plants — or how much — that knowledge is a gift to pass on. And it's especially important today to pass those little seeds of wisdom and knowledge along to children. What we learn to love as children, we will love, respect, and protect as adults. It is these children and this generation that will be the future caretakers of our herbal traditions and the stewards of healing plants. Let's teach them well.

CHAPTER ONE

HERBAL MEDICINE FOR CHILDREN

A long time ago, when I was just a child, my grandmother took me into her gardens and introduced me to her weeds. When we walked in the scented oak forest, she rubbed my skin with fresh bay leaves, assuring me it would prevent poison oak and keep the insects from swarming over us. When I fell in the nettle patches, she soothed the painful welts with the fresh juice of that plant. Her teachings were without fuss. Strong and powerful, like her, her words sank deep and took root in my heart. That magic my grandmother taught me in the garden of my childhood stayed with me throughout my life, and I have continued the journey into the green.

I've studied the healing power of herbs with many gifted teachers, traveled to many regions with rich herbal histories, come to know a great many more plants, and studied the science as well as the art of herbal healing. Still, the things I learned as a child with my grandmother have remained some of the most powerful teachings of my life. It is those simple yet powerful lessons that I seek to pass on to you and your children.

The very act of studying herbs and using plants for health and well-being instills in most people a deep appreciation for Mother Earth and a more balanced way of living. If we teach our children early a love of the earth and a respect for plants and nature, they grow up with a much greater sense of balance and engagement, especially in this age of technology and dissociation from the natural world. In what has been termed a "nature-deficient" society, children especially need and benefit from a close association with plants and the great outdoors. The ancient system of healing with plants is one of the practical and eminently useful ways we can connect deeply with nature. And when we learn to connect with nature as children, it's a lesson we carry with us for life.

USING HERBS FOR CHILDREN'S HEALTH CARE

NOT ONLY DO HERBS SERVE as wonderful teachers for our children, but they also provide an effective, gentle system of healing for them. Children's bodies are sensitive and respond naturally and quickly to the healing energy of herbs. Administered wisely, herbs do not upset the delicate ecological balance of children's small bodies (as does much of modern medicine) but rather work in harmony with their systems.

Contrary to popular opinion, herbs and orthodox medicine are not at odds; they are two systems of healing that can complement one another. Herbs work wonderfully to help resolve the simple aches and ailments of everyday life, to nourish the body so that it's better able to ward off and fight infection, and to help restore constitutional wellness. Allopathic medicine, in turn, is a superior system for life-threatening illness, when acute symptoms need to be brought under control rapidly.

Though allopathic medicine can work quickly, effectively, and efficiently, it is single-minded in its healing approach: get rid of the symptoms quickly before they do harm. Unfortunately, as we are learning, the harm is often in the medicine itself. Pharmaceutical medications are strong, especially so in the small bodies of children, and can have unhelpful side effects. So, of course, use pharmaceuticals when necessary, but whenever possible, rely instead on gentle, time-tested herbal remedies. Herbal medicine is not only effective but also ecologically sane (not polluting the waterways and soil as modern drugs are known to do) and cost effective (you can even grow much of your own medicine!).

If you intend to use both herbal and allopathic medicines in caring for yourself and your family, make sure your doctor or health care provider is familiar with both systems, and consult with him or her whenever you're in doubt about whether it's appropriate to use herbs and pharmaceuticals together. The herbs mentioned in this particular book have no unwelcome interactions with pharmaceuticals; they are gentle and safe to use even with very young children. But if you progress to using other herbs and natural remedies, you may want a knowledgeable holistic health care provider as a guide.

When to Use Herbs

Herbs can be used with confidence for simple ailments such as colic, rashes, teething, and everyday bumps and bruises, as well as the many common illnesses that children often contract, such as ear infections, colds and flu, stomach bugs, and chicken pox. Herbs can also be used as supplements to allopathic medicine when dealing with more complicated health problems.

If herbal remedies don't give the results you were hoping for, then consider allopathic treatment as the next step.

When to Seek Medical Help

Allopathic medicine is an excellent emergency- or crisis-oriented system, and it is by far the best system of medicine for serious and life-threatening situations. Be sure to establish a relationship with a pediatrician, preferably one who is holistically minded, while your child is well so you'll be prepared if ever there is a situation that requires medical attention.

Seek medical help if the child:

- Is not responding to the herbal treatments you are using.
- Shows signs of serious illness, such as acute fever greater than 102°F/39°C, low-grade persistent fever, hemorrhaging, delirium, severe dizziness, unconsciousness, or severe abdominal pain.
- Is lethargic and weak, unresponsive, or difficult to awaken.
- Complains of a stiff neck and headache and is unable to touch his or her chin to the chest. Or, in babies, the fontanel (soft spot on top of the head) may bulge. These are possible early signs of meningitis, which requires immediate medical attention.
- Contracts recurring ear infections.
- Has difficulty breathing or turns blue around the lips.
- Becomes dehydrated. Warning signs are dry lips, dry mouth, and absence of urination over 6 hours.
- Shows signs of a severe allergic reaction, particularly after a bee sting or ingestion of a new food. Warning signs include difficulty breathing or swallowing, flushing or redness of the face, swelling of the face or tongue, nausea or vomiting, severe abdominal pain, palpitations, anxiety, or other unusual responses.
- Has red streaks on the skin emanating from a point of infection; this could indicate blood poisoning.
- Has a severe burn, a burn extending over an area twice the size of the child's hand, or any burn that appears to be infected.

GETTING PERSPECTIVE ON THE SAFETY OF HERBS

Interestingly, parents are often willing to use herbs themselves, and they are even comfortable recommending them to others, but when it comes to their children, they become hesitant. While herbal remedies can be just as effective as pharmaceuticals in many cases, as well as being safer, with fewer side effects, parents often choose allopathic medication because "that's what the doctor ordered," and when it comes to the health of their children they're reluctant to look outside the traditional medical establishment.

How safe are pharmaceuticals? The American Association of Poison Control Centers reports that every year in the United States there are over 1,500 accidental deaths from legally prescribed prescription drugs, making them the fourth leading cause of death in the nation. Add the astonishing 1,000-plus deaths caused by the side effects of drugs and we have a whopping 2,500 medication-related deaths per year.

What about herbs? How many calls does the AAPCC get about them? According to recent statistics, the AAPCC gets so few calls about poisoning from herbs and herbal remedies that they don't even have a special category for herbs.

Thankfully, we don't have to choose between the two systems of medicine. Both traditional herbal medicine and modern allopathic medicine offer tremendous gifts of healing, and each system complements the other. Together they form a comprehensive system of health and healing, each having strengths and weaknesses. But knowing when to choose herbs and when to choose pharmaceutical medications is paramount.

Idiosyncratic Reactions

Herbs are among the safest medications available on earth. This does not mean that there are not toxic plants or herbal remedies that can cause harmful reactions. But the herbs we use today have been used for centuries by people around the world, so we have a pretty good idea of how they work on the human body and the reactions they cause. (And, again, this book includes only the safest herbs that have had a long history of use.)

....

The Patch Test

Some children are more prone to allergies than others. If you're worried about how your child will react to a particular herb, try a patch test. Make a tea with the herb (see instructions on pages 95–97), and then "paint" a small amount of the tea onto the skin of your child's inner arm. Wait 24 hours, keeping an eye on that spot. If you notice any adverse reactions — skin rash, itchy eyes, throat swelling, itchiness — discontinue use immediately.

If the child does not experience an adverse reaction, have him or her drink a very small amount of the tea. Again, wait 24 hours. Discontinue if any signs of allergic reaction appear.

If your child does have a reaction to an herb, to rule out the possibility of another cause for the symptoms, you may wish to try the herb again, prepared in the same manner and administered in the same amount, after a few days. If the child experiences discomfort again, then you can attribute the effects to the herb and look for another, more compatible herb.

....

Occasionally an herb will stimulate an idiosyncratic reaction in an individual. This doesn't make the herb toxic; it's just a poor choice for that particular individual. For example, strawberries, a perfectly delicious fruit, are sweet nectar to some and noxious to others.

Avoiding the Hysteria: Using Herbs Wisely

There are many reports surfacing these days about the toxicity of herbs. Even perfectly benign substances such as chamomile and peppermint are winding up on the "black list." The reason for this is not that more people are using herbs (as is often suggested), but that people are using herbs in ways that allow more concentrated dosages, far beyond what common sense would dictate. In the past, herbs were most often taken as teas, syrups, and tinctures. These preparations contain modest dosages of the whole herb. Herb capsules, which pack large volumes of herb into small pills, allow for huge dosages, while standardized preparations contain supremely concentrated extracts of particular plant constituents — *not* the whole plant — that range far beyond the normal concentrations found in nature. These types of concentrated dosages have not been available until recently.

With not centuries but millennia of experience behind the use of medicinal herbs, you can be assured of their safety for your child — indeed, for your whole family. But be a wise practitioner of herbal remedies:

- Use only those herbs that have a record of safety.
- Follow the appropriate dosages outlined in this book.
- Discontinue use of an herb if you suspect it to be the cause of an idiosyncratic response.
- Whenever you're in doubt or when your child isn't responding to herbal remedies, consult with your holistic health care professional.

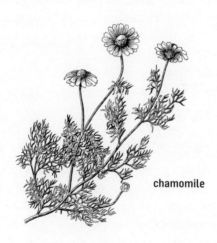

chamomile

CHAPTER TWO

THE BEST HERBS FOR CHILDREN

Almost any herb that is safe for an adult is safe for a child as long as the dosage is adjusted to account for the lesser size and weight of the child. That being said, herbs that are more gentle in action are better suited to the more sensitive constitution of children.

The herbs listed in this chapter are the ones most often recommended for children. They are generally recognized as being safe and benign, with no residual buildup or side effects in the body. These "gentle" herbs can be very powerful and effective, but they act in a less abrasive manner than other stronger-acting medicinal herbs or pharmaceuticals. These herbs generally strengthen the immune system, fortify the nervous system, and in a multitude of ways support the body's innate ability to heal itself. They should form the foundation of herbal health care for children.

Anise (*Pimpinella anisum*)

PARTS USED: primarily the seeds, but the leaves are also useful

BENEFITS: Anise has a long history of being used as a medicinal herb and culinary spice and has been cultivated for over 4,000 years. It is primarily used as a carminative (gas-expelling), warming digestive aid. It can also be helpful in treating mild urinary infections and as an expectorant (helps expel mucus) in respiratory ailments. It has a tasty licorice-like flavor that most children enjoy.

SUGGESTED USES: Use as a tea for colic and other digestive problems. Because of its sweet flavor, anise is often blended with less tasty herbs to make them more palatable. It makes a tasty syrup.

Astragalus (*Astragalus membranaceus*)

PART USED: roots

BENEFITS: Adaptogenic (resistance-building) and toning, astragalus sometimes is called the young person's ginseng. While echinacea supports the immune system's first line of defense, astragalus strengthens the deep immune system by helping rebuild the bone marrow reserve that regenerates the body's protective shield. Numerous studies have shown its effectiveness in helping young children through chemotherapy and radiation therapy.

SUGGESTED USES: Astragalus is best used in tea for helping patients overcome long-term illness and low energy and to help support and build immunity. The root looks exactly like the tongue depressors doctors use, and children may enjoy chewing on it, just like a licorice stick. You can incorporate it into soups and broths; just place a root or two (whole or chopped) in the pot and simmer for several hours.

Catnip (*Nepeta cataria*)

PARTS USED: leaves and flowers

BENEFITS: While catnip sends cats into spasms of pleasure, it is an excellent calming herb for people and is used to relieve all manner of stress. It is particularly beneficial for lowering fever and relieving the pain of teething. It is also a restorative digestive aid used to relieve indigestion, diarrhea, and colic. Catnip is highly recommended for children, as it is calming, relaxing, pain relieving, and gentle.

SUGGESTED USES: Serve as a tea throughout the day to alleviate teething pain. Catnip is quite bitter tasting, so combine it with pleasant-tasting herbs such as oats and lemon balm, or mix it with fruit juice to make it more palatable. Give a couple drops of catnip tincture before meals to serve as a digestive aid. A few drops of the tincture before bedtime will help calm a fussy child. This is one of the best herbs to reduce childhood fevers; use as both a tincture and an enema for this purpose.

Chamomile (*Matricaria recutita, Anthemis nobilis*, and related species)

PARTS USED: primarily the flowers, but the leaves are also useful

BENEFITS: This little plant is a healing wonder. In its flowering tops it has rich amounts of an essential oil that acts as a powerful anti-inflammatory agent. The flowers make a wonderfully soothing tea that is good for the nerves and for digestion. It is especially useful for digestive problems caused by stress, including colic.

SUGGESTED USES: Chamomile tea sweetened with honey can be served throughout the day to calm a stressed or nervous child. A massage oil made with chamomile essential oil can be used for similar calming effects, and to soothe sore, achy muscles. A few drops of chamomile tincture will aid digestion; administer before feeding time.

CAUTION: Though chamomile is considered to be generally benign, it is a member of the composite family, and some individuals have allergies to plants in this family. If your child is very sensitive and/or prone to allergies, do a patch test (page 7) before introducing chamomile to him or her.

Using Stronger-Acting Herbs

People often express concern about using stronger-acting medicinal herbs such as goldenseal, valerian, or St. John's wort for children, but I've found them to be extremely useful and effective. However, be sensible: Use stronger-acting herbs in small amounts for short periods of time, and use them in conjunction with the milder herbs profiled here.

Dill (*Anethum graveolens*)

PARTS USED: primarily the seeds, but the leaves are tasty

BENEFITS: Dill's name comes from *dilla*, an old Norse word that means "to lull," and it has a fairly strong reputation for being calming and comforting for infants and children. Dill is a good digestive aid, and it has an even greater reputation for expelling gas. It is one of the most well-known herbs for relieving gastric stress, colic, and nervous digestion in children. Dill is a good source of manganese, magnesium, and iron, and contains calcium as well.

SUGGESTED USES: Dill is common as a culinary herb. It is also quite tasty brewed in tea, either alone or with other herbs.

Echinacea (*Echinacea angustifolia*, *E. purpurea*, and related species)

PARTS USED: roots, leaves, flowers, and seeds

BENEFITS: Echinacea works by increasing macrophage T-cell activity, thereby bolstering the body's first line of defense against infection. It is one of our most important immune-stimulating and infection-fighting herbs. Though potent and effective, it is also safe to use for children and has no known side effects or residual buildup.

SUGGESTED USES: Echinacea works best when taken not every day but at the onset of infection or when precautions are warranted (i.e., everyone at daycare is sick — keep your child home and give her echinacea!). At the first sign of a cold or flu, give echinacea in tea or tincture form to boost immunity and help ward off the infection. It works best if taken in frequent but small doses; for instance, adults would take ½ teaspoon of tincture or ¼ cup of tea every 30 to 40 minutes, with the dosage adjusted accordingly for a child (see page 92). It is also useful as a tea or tincture for children's respiratory and bronchial infections, and it can be used in a spray to soothe sore throats. For sore gums and mouth inflammation, use the tea or diluted tincture as a mouthwash, flavored with peppermint or spearmint essential oil.

While echinacea is most effective taken internally, it can also be used as a wash or poultice externally to treat skin infections.

CAUTION: Like chamomile, echinacea is a member of the composite family and may cause an allergic reaction in rare individuals. If your child is very sensitive and/or prone to allergies, do a patch test (page 7) before introducing echinacea to him or her.

Note: Because of the huge demand for this herb, it has been poached mercilessly from its native habitat and is becoming increasingly rare in the wilds, so avoid wild-harvested echinacea. Instead buy from reliable companies that sell cultivated echinacea, ideally *organically* cultivated. Better yet, grow your own.

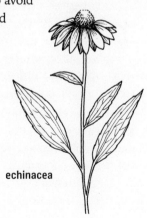

echinacea

Elder *(Sambucus nigra)*

PARTS USED: berries and flowers

BENEFITS: If you travel through Europe during flu season, you'll find a variety of elderberry products lining the pharmacy shelves. Though every part of the plant has its uses, it's the deep blue berries that are my favorite. High in both vitamin A and C, the berries play a key role in the health of the immune system. They also contain significant amounts of flavonoids and anthocyanins that are both heart-protective and immune-enhancing. And the berries (as well as the flowers) contain important antiviral properties. Though it's most often targeted to colds and flu, elder is also useful for upper respiratory infections. It is often combined with echinacea in remedies to support the immune system.

SUGGESTED USES: Elderberries make some of the best syrup you'll ever taste — and it's even effective as medicine, too (see page 74). Elderberries also make a colorful and tasty immune-stimulating tea (it will need to be sweetened or mixed with fruit juice to appeal to most children). The flowers are often used in teas for reducing fever.

CAUTION: There are several varieties of elder; use the type that produces blue, not red, flowers. The red elder is mildly toxic. Berries of the blue elder should be eaten cooked, not raw, as the seeds contain a mild toxin that can produce gastrointestinal discomfort and even poisoning if eaten raw in large amounts.

Elecampane (*Inula helenium*)

PART USED: roots

BENEFITS: Elecampane is a powerful yet gentle expectorant (expels mucus from the lungs and congestion from the respiratory system) and is helpful for treating coughs, bronchitis, and chronic lung infections. It is especially effective for coughs when mixed with echinacea, licorice, and/or marsh mallow root. If the cough is particularly spastic or repetitive, add to the mix a little valerian, a muscle relaxant. If a respiratory or bronchial infection isn't responding readily, try treating it with a mixture of elecampane and pleurisy root; this combination is generally effective for even the most tenacious lung infections.

SUGGESTED USES: Elecampane is not particularly delicious tasting, so be creative when preparing it for children. As a tea, it can be mixed with other more tasty herbs such as licorice and/or marsh mallow root. Add a little cinnamon and sweeten with honey or maple syrup. If using the elecampane-pleurisy blend, mix the tinctures together in equal amounts and serve in water, tea, or fruit juice.

Fennel (*Foeniculum vulgare*)

PARTS USED: primarily the seeds, but the leaves and flowers are also used

BENEFITS: A well-known carminative and digestive aid, this licorice-flavored plant is renowned for its ability to increase and enrich the flow of milk in nursing mothers. Fennel is also an effective antacid; it neutralizes excess acid in the stomach and intestines and also clears uric acid from the joints, helping to reduce inflammation and the pain of arthritis. It is an excellent digestive aid, stimulating digestion, regulating appetite, and relieving flatulence.

SUGGESTED USES: Fennel makes a wonderfully tasty tea for treating colic, improving digestion, and expelling gas from the system. Nursing mothers can drink two to four cups of tea daily to increase and enrich their milk flow. It is also effective in treating eye inflammation and conjunctivitis; use a wash of warm fennel tea that has been strained well through a fine-mesh strainer. Because of its sweet licorice-like flavor, fennel is often blended with other less flavorful herbs to make them more palatable.

Hawthorn (*Crataegus oxyacantha*, *C. monogyna*, and related species)

PARTS USED: fruits, flowers, leaves, and young twigs

BENEFITS: Rich in antioxidants, hawthorn helps build a healthy immune system. It is considered a superior heart tonic, strengthening and nourishing the heart. Hawthorn is outstanding both as a preventive to keep the heart healthy and as a remedy to treat heart disease, edema, angina, and arrhythmia. It is also useful during times of grief and can help us weather the sad times of life.

Though generally thought of as an herb for those with heart issues and/or the elderly, hawthorn is an excellent herb for the children as well. It nourishes the blood, strengthens the immune system, supports good vision, and can help a child get through a time of loss and sadness.

SUGGESTED USES: Hawthorn is tasty when made into a sweetened syrup or jam. It also makes a nice-tasting tea when formulated with other herbs such as hibiscus, oats, and lemon balm. It is quite astringent tasting, so it may have to be sweetened. Or, of course, you could always use in tincture form.

Hibiscus (*Hibiscus sabdariffa* and related species)

PART USED: flowers

BENEFITS: Hibiscus flower is high in vitamin C, bioflavonoids, and antioxidants. It is helpful in restoring and maintaining overall health, supporting immune function, and warding off colds and flus. Because of its high bioflavonoid and vitamin C content, it is also useful for treating mild anemia and poor circulation. With its bright red coloring, hibiscus flower is not just lovely to look at but an excellent source of anthocyanins, which support vascular health. The flower has been used throughout North Africa to maintain respiratory health and is used in a variety of ways to treat respiratory infections and sore throat. Aside from all of this, hibiscus tea is one of the most lovely natural beverages and children generally adore it.

SUGGESTED USES: The large hibiscus flowers make a beautiful ruby red tea. The flavor is somewhat tart, with a sweet aftertaste; children may prefer to have it sweetened. Try making hibiscus flowers into a thick syrup (see page 101), and add this bright red syrup to sparkling water. It's delicious and refreshing, not to mention healthy!

Lemon balm (*Melissa officinalis*)

PART USED: leaves

BENEFITS: Calming, antiviral, and antiseptic, this beautifully fragrant member of the mint family is one of nature's best nervine herbs. It is used as a mild sedative for times of depression and grief, and it is one of the most important natural antiviral plants known. It is especially useful for recurrent outbreaks of herpes, shingles, and thrush and will serve as a preventive if taken on a regular basis.

SUGGESTED USES: Though lemon balm dries well, its flavor is best fresh. It can be tinctured or encapsulated, but because of its refreshing pleasant flavor, lemon balm is most often served as a tea. The tea can be served with lemon and honey throughout the day to alleviate stress and anxiety, and also as a preventive for herpes, shingles, and thrush (all related viral infections). It is an important remedy for any viral infection, including measles and mumps. For a delicious nervine tonic tea, blend equal amounts of lemon balm, oats, and chamomile. To support a person during a time of grief, add hawthorn to this blend. Add St. John's wort to the blend to treat mild to moderate depression. Fresh lemon balm makes an excellent syrup (see page 101), which can be added to sparkling water for a refreshing spritzer or all-natural soda.

lemon balm

Licorice (*Glycyrrhiza glabra*)

PART USED: roots

BENEFITS: Licorice is rich in antiviral properties, making it an excellent remedy for any viral infection, including herpes, shingles, thrush, measles, and mumps. It is often combined with lemon balm for this purpose. Its high mucilaginous content and antiviral and anti-inflammatory properties make it a soothing and healing remedy for sore throats, respiratory infections, viral infections, and gastrointestinal inflammations such as ulcers. It also has mild laxative properties that can help with mild cases of constipation.

SUGGESTED USES: Licorice is very sweet and is often combined with other herbs to make them more palatable. On the other hand, licorice root by itself is often *too* sweet and so is blended with other herbs to tone the sweetness down. Licorice makes an excellent syrup (see page 101), which can be added to sparkling water for a tasty soda. Children enjoy chewing on licorice sticks, and you can even give a "stick" of licorice root to a teething baby to chew on — though you may have to give the root a few "chews" yourself to soften it enough that the young one can begin to chew on it. It can usually keep the teething baby busy for a little while, at least.

CAUTION: Though most children don't suffer from these ailments, licorice should not be used by those with hypertension or kidney/bladder problems, by anyone undergoing steroid therapy, or by anyone who is taking medication for a heart or kidney ailment.

Marsh mallow (*Althaea officinalis*)

PARTS USED: primarily the roots, but the leaves and flowers are also useful

BENEFITS: Marsh mallow can be used like slippery elm as a soothing, cooling demulcent in herbal remedies, and it is much more readily available and easy to grow. Marsh mallow root has both antibacterial and anti-inflammatory properties. It is especially soothing to inflamed, irritated membranes and is often used in tea blends and tinctures for sore throat, respiratory infections, and digestive irritation.

SUGGESTED USES: Serve as a tea for sore throat, digestive irritation, bronchial inflammation, or diarrhea or constipation. Marsh mallow is very soothing to the urinary tract and is often recommended for urinary tract and bladder infections. It also has external applications: Mix it with water into a thick paste to soothe burns and irritated skin, or combine it with oatmeal as a soothing wash or bath for irritated, itchy dry skin.

Nettle (*Urtica dioica*)

PARTS USED: primarily the fresh leaves and young tops, but the roots and seeds are also used

BENEFITS: Nettle is a treasure trove of vitamins and minerals. It is an especially good source of iron and calcium and is used to help restore these two important minerals in pregnant and nursing mothers (for this purpose mix it with raspberry leaf, another good nutritive and also a female reproductive tonic). The calcium in nettle is found in an easy-to-assimilate biochelated form, which makes it especially helpful for relieving stress and nerve repair. It is especially healing for nerves when paired with green milky oats. Nettle is also valuable for its role in supporting tissue and bone repair and is often blended with oats and horsetail for this purpose. Because of its high calcium and mineral content, it helps support dense bone growth and can help alleviate growing pains in young children. It is also an effective remedy for allergies and hay fever; it has been known to work wonders for some people. Nettle root is a renowned herb for men and supports prostate and sexual health.

SUGGESTED USES: Nettle tastes similar to spinach and is often steamed, sprinkled with olive oil, lemon juice, and a little feta, and served as a mineral-rich side dish at meals. It can be used in place of spinach or other steamed greens in any recipe. However, it must be steamed completely and thoroughly; if undercooked, it will "sting." The small hairs located on the underside of the nettle leaf and on the stems are filled with formic acid, the same substance in bee stings, which causes skin to swell and results in a painful, itchy rash. Pick nettles with gloves, be careful not to brush up against it, and teach your children to respect this plant. If anyone does happen to get "stung," apply a plantain leaf poultice to draw the toxins out.

Though nettle can be used as a tincture or tea for allergies, it seems most effective for this purpose in freeze-dried form. When possible, combined capsules of freeze-dried nettle with nettle tea and/or tincture for an even more profound effect.

Oats (*Avena sativa*)

PARTS USED: oats and stalks

BENEFITS: Green milky oats are considered among the best nutritive tonics for the nervous system and are recommended during cases of nervous exhaustion, stress, and overall irritation and grumpiness. The milky oats are good sources of silica, calcium, and have mucilaginous properties. They are especially recommended for imbalances of the nervous system.

SUGGESTED USES: Both the milky green oats and oat stalks make a tasty tea, either alone or blended with other herbs such as lemon balm, hawthorn, and hibiscus. It is delicious when brewed double to triple strength and then mixed with fruit juice. Oat tea is recommended for children who are nervous, hyperactive, and stressed and/or are constantly agitated or irritated. Because of its rich mucilaginous content, oatmeal baths are wonderfully soothing for dry itchy skin and for skin irritations.

Milky Oats

For medicinal purposes, herbalists prefer green milky oats, harvested before they are fully ripened. They're called "milky" because when you press on the oats, tiny droplets of milk shoot out. However, the fully ripe oats also have their uses. Oatmeal, made from the ripe oats, is both nutritive and soothing, and it makes an excellent meal for those recovering from illness. Oatmeal baths (see page 70) are recommended for dry, itchy skin and for skin irritation.

Peppermint (*Mentha piperita*)

PARTS USED: leaves and flowers

BENEFITS: Peppermint is a blast of pure green energy. It's not that there aren't stronger stimulants, but few make you feel as renewed and refreshed as peppermint. Peppermint is often added to brain tonic formulas. It is also commonly used as a digestive aid and is effective for easing nausea and stomach cramps.

SUGGESTED USES: Use for children when they have tummy aches or sluggish digestion, or when they just need a little radiant energy. Peppermint can be made into a tea, tincture (diluted), and mouthwash. It also makes a delicious syrup, which can be added to sparkling water for a cooling drink. I like to introduce children to this plant in the garden and often have them nibble its refreshing, tasty leaves. The essential oil of peppermint is also very healing and useful; however, because of its concentration, be careful with it, especially when using it with children. A drop of the essential oil added to a little water makes a refreshing and stomach-settling mouthwash for a child who's experiencing a bout of vomiting and helps clear the mouth of foul taste.

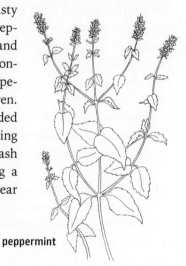

peppermint

Red clover (*Trifolium pratense*)

PARTS USED: flowering top and leaves

BENEFITS: One of the best respiratory tonics, red clover is traditionally used with children who have chronic chest complaints — frequent coughs, colds, and other respiratory issues. Red clover is exceptionally rich in minerals, most notably calcium, nitrogen, and iron. It is one of the traditional "blood purifiers" used to treat conditions of the blood, heart, and liver. It is useful for all skin conditions, including psoriasis, eczema, and dry itchy skin.

SUGGESTED USES: Use red clover to make a delicious sweet-flavored tea. Blend it with other respiratory tonic herbs such as mullein and elecampane to treat persistent respiratory problems. Red clover combines well with oats and lemon balm for treating skin disorders and with hawthorn and hibiscus for treating blood and heart issues. As a blood purifier, red clover tea or tincture is recommended in cases of congestion or growths on or in the body, such as cysts, tumors, and fibroids. It is also helpful in alleviating hay fever and allergies and is often combined with nettle for this purpose.

CAUTION: Do not use red clover with those who are taking blood-thinning medication, hemophiliacs, or those who bleed heavily, as it can potentially exacerbate the problem.

Red raspberry (*Rubus idaeus*)

PARTS USED: leaves, young shoots, and fruits

BENEFITS: Raspberry leaf has a long history of use as a reproductive tonic for both men and women. It also helps reduce excessive menstruation and vaginal bleeding and is a renowned tonic for women during pregnancy and childbirth. Raspberry leaves are rich in vitamins and minerals, particularly calcium and iron, which makes them especially valuable for pregnant and nursing mothers, infants, and children. The leaves are often blended with other nutritive herbs such as nettle, oats, and red clover as a tonic tea for pregnant and nursing moms.

SUGGESTED USES: Because of its astringent properties, raspberry leaf as a tea or tincture is helpful for relieving diarrhea and dysentery. Raspberry leaf mixed with white oak bark and/or spilanthes is an effective mouthwash for sore or infected gums.

Rose (*Rosa canina* and related species)

PARTS USED: primarily the seeds (rose hips), but the leaves and flowers are also used

BENEFITS: Rose hips contain more vitamin C than almost any other herb, and many times the amount found in citrus fruit. Vitamin C is a noted antioxidant with disease-fighting capabilities. Rose leaves are astringent and toning and are often used in cosmetic recipes. The flowers are used in many medicinal formulas as well as in love potions and flower essences.

SUGGESTED USES: Make fresh rose hips into a vitamin-rich syrup or jam. Dried seedless rose hips also make a delicious raw jam that is *so* easy to make (see the recipe on the next page). Rose hips also make a much loved, mild and sweet tea.

rose

HOW TO MAKE ROSE HIP JAM

This raw rose hip jam is simple to make and doesn't involve any cooking at all. It's so straightforward that young children can easily make it on their own — and usually love doing so! The trick is to start with dried deseeded rose hips, which you can buy from most herb shops. (You can deseed and dry your own rose hips, but it is a timely process.) Then follow these steps:

Step 1. Fill a pint jar half full of dried deseeded rose hips.

Step 2. Fill the jar three-quarters full with apple juice or cider, covering the rose hips with an inch or two of the liquid.

Step 3. Put a lid on the jar and let it sit at room temperature for several hours or overnight. The rose hips will absorb the juice and become thick and jam-like.

Step 4. Usually this jam doesn't require any further sweetening, but if necessary, add a teaspoon or so of maple syrup or honey. You can also add ground cinnamon and other tasty herbs to enhance the flavor if you wish. But I love it just the way it is — deliciously plain and simple.

Step 5. Store in a glass jar with tight-fitting lid in the refrigerator, where it will keep for 2 to 3 weeks. Let your children eat this jam by the spoonful!

Slippery elm (*Ulmus fulva, U. rubra*)

PART USED: inner bark

BENEFITS: The soft, mucilaginous inner bark of *Ulmus fulva*, the slippery elm tree, is one of the most useful remedies for soothing any and all inflammation, internal or external. It is particularly valuable for burns, sore throats, respiratory infections, and digestive problems. It is also useful for soothing the inflammation caused by diarrhea and constipation. It is still commonly found in lozenges to soothe sore and irritated throats.

SUGGESTED USES: The sweet flavor of slippery elm combines well with licorice, fennel, and cinnamon and makes a tasty, soothing throat and digestive tea. To make the tea, soak the bark in cold or cool water overnight, or simmer for 10 to 15 minutes. Powdered slippery elm can be added to oatmeal to make a very soothing, easily digested, and healing gruel for those who are debilitated or ill. The powder is also easily mixed into medicinal "candy balls" (see page 98). Or you can make "syrup" of sorts: Combine 1 tablespoon powdered slippery elm, 1 teaspoon ground cinnamon, 1 cup warm water, and 1 tablespoon honey. Blend well in a blender. This syrup will be thick; adults generally dislike the slimy texture, but children often love it! Use as a cough medicine and to help restore health after illness.

CAUTION: It was a dilemma whether to include slippery elm in this chapter because it is currently on the United Plant Savers at-risk list (see page 119). But when nothing else does the trick, a small amount of slippery elm powder may ease a child's swollen sore throat or digestive issues, or help build up health in a child who's been sick for an extended period. Just use it sparingly, only as needed. Whenever possible, use another herb with similar properties, such as marsh mallow root. And buy only farm-grown or ethically harvested (from fallen limbs) slippery elm.

Spearmint (*Mentha spicata*)

PARTS USED: leaves and flowers

BENEFITS: Cooling, refreshing, and uplifting, spearmint is one of the most popular mints. Children often appreciate spearmint more than peppermint, as spearmint is a bit milder. It makes a delicious and refreshing tea, useful for lifting a person's mood and brightening the spirits.

SUGGESTED USES: Use spearmint to "sweeten" the stomach and breath after sickness, especially vomiting. Just add a drop of the essential oil to water or brew a cup of fresh tea and use it to rinse the mouth several times. Spearmint makes a lovely syrup, which can be added to sparkling water for a light, uplifting drink; it's also wonderful in iced tea, as are the fresh leaves.

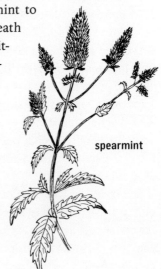

spearmint

The fresh leaves can be added to honey to make spearmint honey: Layer a few inches of fresh spearmint leaves on the bottom of a pint jar. Pour warmed honey over the leaves. Put on a lid and let sit in a warm, sunny window for several days, or until the honey has the scent and taste of spearmint. You can scoop the leaves out or leave them in the honey. Use this honey as an "instant tea" by adding a spoonful or two to hot water. Or use the honey to sweeten and flavor other teas.

Stevia (*Stevia rebaudiana*)

PART USED: leaves

BENEFITS: Stevia is really a miracle herb. Fifty times sweeter than sugar, it has no calories, doesn't cause tooth decay, and is useful in the treatment of both hypoglycemia and hyperglycemia — it not only sweetens but helps normalize blood sugar levels. Furthermore, stevia is a remedy for pancreatic imbalances and can be used by most diabetics without causing sugar-related issues.

SUGGESTED USES: Because stevia is so intensely sweet, it has to be blended with other herbs to be palatable. If more than 2 percent is added to a tea blend, it will usually dominate the flavor, so be sparing when using it. Children, however, who love the intensely sweet flavor of stevia, are often found "grazing" on it!

Wild cherry (*Prunus serotina*)

PART USED: inner bark

BENEFITS: Wild cherry bark is among the most well-known cough remedies and expectorants and is one of the few herbs still included in the United States Pharmacopeia's annual drug reference. It can still be found in many commercial cough remedies. It also improves digestion and promotes healthy bowel function.

SUGGESTED USES: Wild cherry is a favorite herb in teas, syrups, and tinctures for coughs and colds. Mix it with elderberries for their powerful antiviral and immune-enhancing properties. Mix it with elecampane for those tenacious lingering coughs. For deep bronchial infection, mix wild cherry bark with elecampane and pleurisy root; this triple-powered blend will heal most deep-seated bronchial infections.

CAUTION: In order not to harm the beautiful trees, collect the soft inner bark from fallen limbs after a storm. Never debark around the trunk of a tree or it will die.

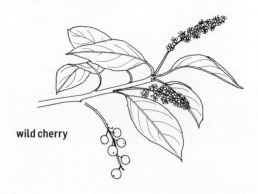

wild cherry

CHAPTER THREE

TREATING COMMON CHILDHOOD AILMENTS

By closely observing your child, you can usually detect when he or she is stressed, anxious, or out of balance, and thus more susceptible to illness. Illness rarely just occurs by chance; generally it is the result of a taxed immune system, emotional imbalance, lack of sleep, poor hygiene, poor nutrition, or allergies. Sometimes illness occurs because the child is just having too much fun whirling through life. Children live in passion and excitement much of the time and the energy required to maintain such high levels of activity can leave even the most exuberant of spirits exhausted and depleted.

All children are born with inherent strengths and weaknesses. Watch for these patterns early in life. If health and wellness issues are noted and addressed at a young age, they can often be corrected and become strengths rather than weaknesses as the child grows older. However, if left unattended, these childhood problems sometimes develop into chronic illnesses that plague a person for his or her whole life. So pay close attention to the ebb and flow of your child's energy levels. Observe your child through the seasons, noting which season brings which special health challenges. Note which types of illnesses your child seems most susceptible to. This will help you become more aware of your child's health patterns and empower and enable you and your child to be a step ahead — to focus on wellness rather than illness.

The remedies and therapies shared in this chapter will help you and your family get through all the typical ailments of childhood with as much grace, resiliency, and immune-building support — and, sometimes just as important, sleep — as possible. Please note that it is meant to complement, not replace, the professional advice of your family health care provider. If at any time your child continues to get worse, rather than better, please consult with your pediatrician.

TEETHING

UNAVOIDABLY, TEETHING AFFECTS all children, with varying degrees of discomfort. Though not an illness, it generally is a time of great frustration for both parent and child — for parents because it seems no matter how hard they try they can't help their child feel better, and for the child because he or she is experiencing one of the early pains of life, and it hurts!

Teething can give rise to various symptoms. Intermittent fever, diaper and other rashes, extreme crankiness, and diarrhea are not uncommon. Treat each symptom appropriately, following the guidelines suggested in this book, but remember that support is the primary lesson called for here. The teething process is natural, like many of the other life cycles we all go through in a lifetime. It marks the child's first experience of "biting in," her ability to deal with the stress of life, to call on her own powers as well as the support of family and friends. Thousands of human babies have gone through this before, and yours can too. The rewards will be a shining set of healthy teeth and the ability to enjoy another of life's great pleasures: good eating.

On the following pages are some of my favorite herbal remedies for teething problems.

Catnip Tea

This is an old standby for both child and parent during the teething times. Catnip is soothing to the nervous system and helps relieve acute pain as well as teething-related fever. Administer as tea or tincture in frequent small doses (dilute the tincture in warm water). The tea itself is not tasty, so you may have to be creative to get your child to drink it. Try formulating catnip with other gentle, better-tasting nervines such as chamomile, rose, passionflower, or lemon balm. Or mix it with apple juice and freeze into herbal popsicles. You can also make a strong tea, soak a clean wet cloth in it, then place the cloth in the freezer; when it's almost frozen but still soft enough to chew, let your child chew on this "teething rag."

The famed 19th-century herb doctor Dr. Jethro Kloss, in his equally famous book *Back to Eden*, noted that if every mother had catnip tea on her shelf, she would save herself "many sleepless nights and doctor's bills, and also save the baby much suffering." It was particularly thoughtful of him to consider the mother, and following his advice, I always suggest a blend of catnip, lemon balm, and passionflower tea for the parents of teething children.

Calcium-Rich Tea

A high-calcium blend is very helpful to give to a child throughout the teething period. It is most effective if it is given several weeks or even months before teething begins. Calcium supports healthy bone, tissue, and ligament growth, and it also soothes and calms the nervous system.

High-Calcium Tea

An excellent blend of herbs that add high-quality, naturally biochelated calcium and other important minerals to the diet, High-Calcium Tea is also helpful for children during growth spurts or when recovering from bone or muscle injury.

2 parts lemon balm leaf
2 parts green milky oats
2 parts rose hips
1 part nettle leaf
1 part raspberry leaf
½ part cinnamon bark
¼ part horsetail leaf
Pinch of stevia leaf to sweeten (optional)

1. Combine the herbs and store in an airtight container.

2. To use, prepare as an infusion, following the directions on page 96. Administer according to the child's size and age, following the dosage guidelines beginning on page 91.

raspberry

Rose Hip Syrup or Jam

Rose hips are mildly anti-inflamatory, and frequent doses of rose hip syrup or rose hip jam can often relieve teething symptoms. As a rich source of vitamin C, rose hips also support immune health during this stressful time in the baby's life. Give four to six drops of rose hip syrup, or a small spoonful of rose hip jam, every hour for infants. For older children give 100 to 200 mg vitamin C in acerola tablets daily along with frequent teaspoon doses of rose hip syrup or jam. To make the syrup, follow the directions on page 101; to make the jam, see the recipe on page 28.

Hyland's Teething (and Colic) Tablets

Hyland's makes a wonderful homeopathic teething tablet for children. Interestingly, many parents have reported that although Hyland's teething formula works well, the company's formula for colic is even more effective for teething babies. So I generally recommend Hyland's colic formula for teething difficulties. Try both and see which works best for you.

Herbal Pops

Frozen pops of catnip or chamomile tea are excellent for teething children to suck on. The cold helps numb the gums and relieves the pain, while the herbs are calming. Children generally love these pops and will suck on them intently until the pain subsides and they're gurgling happily again. You can mix the tea with apple juice before freezing if that will help encourage your child to enjoy it.

COLIC

COLIC CAN BE A HEART-WRENCHING experience for both the parents and the infant. It is generally caused by painful spasmodic contractions of the infant's immature digestive tract or by air and gas trapped in the intestines. The digestive tract of an infant generally takes about three months to mature. Most cases of colic clear up within this time period, though some persist longer.

The following suggestions are all gentle and effective and work in harmony with the sensitive nature of the infant.

Create a Relaxed Environment

Often colicky children are extremely sensitive to their environment. Since you, the parent, are your child's primary source of emotional and physical nourishment, your own well-being can contribute to easing colic. Quiet, peaceful music during mealtimes is often helpful. Mothers should drink warm nervine teas such as chamomile, lemon balm, and passionflower before nursing. Feeding time should, whenever possible, be a time of quiet, restful sharing. If you are feeling stressed out and tense, the infant will often respond with similar energy. Of course, this does not mean that all colicky babies have stressed-out parents, but it is important to note that a peaceful environment is conducive to creating well-being for the child.

Avoid Irritating Foods

Nursing mothers should avoid foods that could be irritating to the infant's digestive tract. While every child's system is different, some foods are common irritants. The brassica family, for example, which includes cabbage, broccoli, cauliflower, kale, and collards, is high in sulfur, which creates gas in the intestines and can create discomfort not only in infants but in adults as well. Avoid hot, spicy foods; an infant's system just isn't ready for them yet. And avoid chocolate, peanuts, and foods high in sugar; such foods slow down digestive action, cause congestion in the digestive tract, and add to the spasms and contractions of colic. Consider monitoring your diet and your child's colicky symptoms to determine which foods may be irritating to the baby.

You may also consider giving up coffee, or at least drinking less. Though the amount of caffeine in your daily coffee may not seem very stimulating to you, that's because your system has learned to adapt to it. Coffee is, nonetheless, a powerful stimulant. Your child's young system will respond readily to its stimulating properties and she/he may become nervous, highly excitable, and, as a result, colicky. Coffee is also very acidic and can adversely affect the immature digestive system of the infant, adding to the difficulties.

Supplement with Acidophilus and Other Probiotics

Acidophilus (*Lactobacillus acidophilus*) and other forms of probiotics are highly recommended for infant colic. These bacteria are naturally occurring in the human digestive system, and supplements will help build up these healthy intestinal flora and support the growth of digestive enzymes. There are special acidophilus preparations for children available in most natural foods stores. To treat colic, double the amount suggested on the product label. If the child is eating solid foods and is not lactose-intolerant, include daily servings of yogurt, kefir, and buttermilk, cultured dairy products that contain helpful probiotics, including acidophilus. Some children enjoy sauerkraut and miso, both of which are good sources of probiotics and excellent for restoring beneficial gut flora.

A nursing mother should eat several servings a day of these cultured foods to help her colicky infant.

Treat with Herbs That Aid Digestion

The most helpful herbs for treating colic are slippery elm, fennel, anise, dill, and catnip. Try giving the infant teas of these herbs to relieve the acute symptoms of colic. Or grind them into a powder and add to the infant's food. It may also be helpful for the mother to include these herbs in her diet if she is breastfeeding.

Marsh Mallow Gruel

This gruel (thick tea) is wonderfully soothing and nourishing. Since the herbs are in powdered form, there's no need to strain the gruel. I generally make this recipe with marsh mallow, but if the colic is tenacious and marsh mallow isn't working, try adding one part slippery elm powder.

  2   parts marsh mallow root powder
  ⅛   part cinnamon bark powder
  ⅛   part fennel seed powder
      Maple syrup

1. Combine the marsh mallow, cinnamon, and fennel seed, and store in an airtight container until ready to use.

2. To prepare, combine 1 tablespoon of the herb mixture and 1 cup of water in a pan. Bring to a boil, cover, and cook over low heat for 10–15 minutes. Sweeten to taste with maple syrup.

3. Serve warm. You can mix it with juice or warm cereal if you prefer. Store any extra gruel in the refrigerator. The infant may drink as much of this tea as desired. A nursing mother should drink 3–4 cups daily.

Seed Tea

This seed-based tea helps an infant expel gas and relieves the symptoms of colic.

> 3 parts anise seed
> 3 parts chamomile flower
> 1 part dill seed
> 1 part fennel seed
> ¼ part catnip leaf
> Pinch of stevia leaf to sweeten

1. Mix the ingredients and store in an airtight container until ready to use.

2. To prepare, pour 1 cup boiling water over 1 tablespoon of the herb mixture and let sit, covered, for 45 minutes. Cool and strain.

3. To relieve colic symptoms, give the infant teaspoon dosages every few minutes until the pain eases. This tea may also be an effective colic preventive if given in small doses before feeding time.

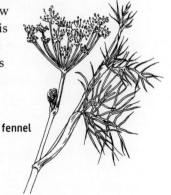

fennel

Colic Tablets

Hyland's has a homeopathic colic tablet that is very good. It is available in most natural foods stores. This safe, all-natural remedy has provided relief for countless colicky babies. Follow the dosages outlined on the bottle.

Old-Fashioned Techniques That Still Work

In the midst of a colic attack, there are a few old-fashioned and effective techniques to try:

- **Herbal bath.** Place your baby in a warm chamomile or lavender bath. If bottle-fed, the baby can enjoy his/her feeding from the comfort of this soothing bath.
- **Herbal compress.** You may be able to help the child's stomach muscles relax by placing a towel that was soaked in warm, calming herb tea — such as chamomile or lavender — over the stomach area. Be certain the towel is adequately warm, but not hot. The combination of warm water and herbal essence will often be just what's needed to relax the child and stop the muscle spasms.
- **Calming essential oil.** If you're trying either the herbal bath or compress mentioned above, a drop or two of lavender or chamomile essential oil in the bathwater or on the towel will often work wonders.

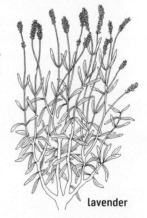

lavender

- **Burping.** And there is always the old reliable burping technique. Pad your shoulder and place the child's head against it. Pat his or her back gently. With regular rhythmic patting, children seem to become hypnotized into forgetting the problem. What is really happening, of course, along with distracting the child from his or her grief for a few moments, is that you are helping to move the gas deposits along.

CRADLE CAP

NEITHER A SERIOUS NOR CONTAGIOUS PROBLEM, cradle cap is a condition that a child will usually outgrow in time. The sebaceous glands of most infants are not developed and may oversecrete, causing a yellowish, oily crust — the "cap" — on a child's scalp. You can remove this buildup and help regulate the activity of the sebaceous glands by gently massaging an herb-infused oil (see the recipe on page 47) into the scalp two or three times daily. Leave the infused oil on overnight, and the next morning the crust can be easily removed by gently massaging. Be sure not to pick at the crust or be too rough with the child's delicate scalp. Shampoo with a mild baby shampoo only when necessary.

Tea for Cradle Cap

If cradle cap continues to be persistent, give the infant this warm herbal tea. These herbs support the lymphatic system and will aid in regulating the sebaceous glands. This tea can also be used as a gentle cleansing wash for the scalp.

> 1 part burdock root, chopped
> 1 part mullein leaf
> 1 part red clover blossom

1. Mix the herbs and store in an airtight container until ready to use.

2. To prepare, pour 1 cup boiling water over 1 teaspoon of the herb mixture and let steep, covered, for 30 minutes. Strain.

3. Give the infant 2 teaspoons of the tea three or four times daily for several weeks.

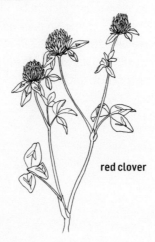

red clover

Cradle Cap Oil

Use this oil on a regular basis to massage the child's scalp. The herbs in this oil blend will gently modulate the sebaceous glands, encouraging them to excrete more efficiently, while the oil will help loosen the cradle cap buildup on the scalp.

    1   part chamomile flower
    1   part mullein leaf
    1   part dried nettle leaf
       Olive oil
       Lavender essential oil

1. Infuse the chamomile, mullein, and nettle in the olive oil, following the instructions on page 111, using the double boiler method and allowing them to steep for 1 hour. Strain, and then add 1 drop of lavender essential oil for each ounce of herbal oil. Bottle, and store in a cool area or the refrigerator.

2. To use, make sure the oil is at room temperature. Gently massage a small amount of the oil into the child's scalp. Gently rub off any excess oil as you finish. Do this two or three times a day.

DIAPER RASH

MOST DIAPER RASHES RESPOND readily to natural therapy. If the diaper rash is persistent or recurrent, or it does not respond to natural therapies, it could be caused by a herpes-related virus or a yeast-related fungus, or it could indicate that the child has an allergy to something she or he is eating or regularly exposed to in the environment. In such cases, consult with your holistic health care practitioner or pediatrician for advice.

One or more of the following irritants generally causes diaper rashes:

- **Harsh detergents.** Laundry detergents can leave a soap residue on cloth diapers. Simply changing to a milder soap can make a difference. Use mild soap flakes such as Ivory or a liquid soap such as pure castile soap. Do not use detergents or ammonia, and never use bleach. As harmful as bleach is for the environment, it is even worse for your baby.

- **Irritating foods.** Certain foods can adversely affect a child's immature digestive system. Spicy foods, citrus fruits, and other high-acid foods are major irritants and can affect the child both when eaten directly and through the mother's milk. Try eliminating these foods from your child's diet (or the nursing mother's diet), and see if that makes a difference.

- **Teething, fever, and other stress-related incidents.** Health stressors cause toxins to be released in the child's system, which can sometimes be manifested as diaper rashes or other skin-related problems. When the incident or event is over, the rash should go away; in the meantime, you can support the child with nurturing, holistic home health care and by treating the symptoms of diaper rash as described here.

Give Acidophilus Preparations

Plant a garden in your belly! Acidophilus and other probiotics help restore healthy gut flora and aid in digestion, assimilation, and elimination. Administer ¼ teaspoon acidophilus culture three times daily. Use a preparation that's formulated especially for children. You can even try spreading acidophilus diluted in plain unsweetened yogurt directly on the rash.

You can also supplement your child's diet with naturally fermented foods like yogurt, kefir, sauerkraut, kimchi, and miso, which contain acidophilus as well as other probiotics that aid in digestion.

Take Off Those Diapers!

When your child has a diaper rash, leave off his or her diapers as much as possible. Let the child be a little nudist. The more exposure to air and sunlight, the better (though of course you must be sure to protect your child's sensitive skin from sunburn and your furniture from frequent watering — and worse).

Apply Herbal Powders

Use plain arrowroot powder or an herbal arrowroot-clay mix for everyday baby powder and as a remedy for diaper rash. Cornstarch, an old-fashioned remedy, is also very effective but is not recommended for use on yeast-related diaper rashes, as it may encourage the growth of certain bacteria. Commercial baby powder is made with talc, which is a possible carcinogen. It also contains synthetic scents, which can be irritating to an infant's sensitive skin. Make your own baby powder (see the recipe below) or buy those that are made with natural ingredients. Take care not to disperse the powder too much around a baby who has respiratory problems.

Baby Powder

This is an excellent daily baby powder. You may wish to lightly scent the powder, but use only pure essential oil and be certain it is nonirritating to the child's sensitive skin. Orange oil is light and refreshing and is often used as the scent for baby powders. Lavender essential oil is another great choice; along with smelling lovely, it has disinfectant properties.

2 parts arrowroot powder

1 part white kaolin or bentonite clay

¼ part comfrey root powder

¼ part marsh mallow root or slippery elm (ethically harvested) powder

A few drops pure essential oil, for scent (optional)

1. Whisk the arrowroot, clay, comfrey, and marsh mallow together. If you're using essential oil, add a few drops, then cover the mixture with a porous cloth or paper towel and let sit for at least a few hours, and up to overnight, so the oils dry. Then whisk again to break up any clots or clumps that might have formed.

2. Place in a shaker bottle, such as a spice jar or a container made for powders. Apply to baby's bottom as needed.

For treating diaper rash: Add to this mixture ⅛ part echinacea powder, ⅛ part goldenseal powder (organically cultivated), and ⅛ part myrrh powder.

For a more serious rash: Mix the powder with water or comfrey tea to form a thin paste. (The paste must be thin; if it's too thick, it can be overly drying to a child's tender skin.) Smooth over the rash and leave on for 30 to 45 minutes. To remove, gently rinse with warm water or soak off in a warm tub. Don't attempt to scrape or peel the paste off or you may further irritate the child's rash.

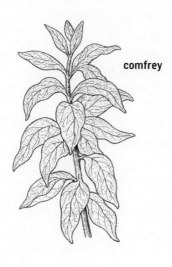

comfrey

Soothing Herbal Salve

An herbal salve made with St. John's wort, comfrey, and calendula (see the recipe below) is one of the best remedies I know of for rashes, scrapes, and other skin irritations. I've been making this formula for more than 25 years, and it is a superior remedy for diaper rashes.

All-Purpose Healing Salve

This is my very favorite salve recipe for diaper rash. It's also useful for soothing and healing cuts, scrapes, burns, and other skin irritations. I prefer to make the salve using a solar-infused oil (see page 113). But if you don't have the time to steep the herbs in olive oil in the sun for 2 weeks, or if there's not much sun, let the herbs steep in a double boiler over very low heat for several hours.

- 1 part calendula flower
- 1 part comfrey leaf
- 1 part St. John's wort flower
- Olive oil
- Grated beeswax
- 1–2 drops essential oil (optional; lavender, tea tree, or chamomile would be a good choice)

1. Prepare the ingredients as a salve, following the instructions on page 115.

2. Apply as needed. To treat diaper rash, wash and dry the baby's bottom after each bowel movement, apply the herbal salve, and follow with a light dusting of baby powder.

This treatment plan used in conjunction with the other suggestions listed on pages 48–51 will generally clear up even the worst diaper rash, unless herpes or staph is involved.

DIARRHEA

THERE ARE FEW CHILDREN WHO have not had a bout of diarrhea — or its counterpart, constipation, which we'll discuss next. Diarrhea can be caused by a number of things, the most common being a reaction to or an excess of certain foods, bacterial or viral infection, teething, fever, or emotional upset.

The primary concern with diarrhea is dehydration, which can occur quickly if fluid intake is inadequate and can be fatal if severe. If your child is having diarrhea, ensure that his or her fluid intake is adequate. Don't just guess: Monitor the amount of liquid the child drinks, and give him or her warm baths, which will help in the absorption of liquid. A warm enema is one of the surest ways to quickly hydrate a young child at risk of dehydration; see pages 109–110 for instructions.

Though liquid intake is essential, it is not necessary that the child eat solid food. It is actually best if she or he consume only liquids, such as herb teas, vegetable broth, and chicken or miso soup. Eating solid food will make the already stressed digestive system work overtime. It also means more runny diapers, as everything eaten will quickly come out. If the child wishes to eat, allow foods such as yogurt, kefir, buttermilk, cottage cheese, potato soup, mashed potatoes (no gravy or butter), and Marsh Mallow Gruel (see recipe on page 42). These foods are easy to digest and will contribute to healing, rather than agitating the digestive system. Though milk products will often exacerbate diarrhea, cultured milk products such as yogurt, kefir, and buttermilk add beneficial bacteria that aid the digestive system. Acidophilus and other probiotics can also help by introducing healthy intestinal flora and boosting the immune system; administer ⅛ teaspoon of acidophilus culture every hour until the diarrhea stops. (Use a supplement formulated for children.) In addition, commercial pediatric electrolyte solutions, such as Pedialyte, are very helpful in preventing dehydration.

Blackberry Root Tincture

A traditional Native American medicinal herb, blackberry root is simply one of the most effective herbs for relieving diarrhea. Along with a high fluid intake, herbal baths, and a very simple diet, this tincture should help remedy the problem. Unfortunately, as common as blackberry is, blackberry root tincture is hard to find. You may have to make your own. Although actually having to dig the root is difficult, you'll find that the tincture itself is easy to make.

> 1 part blackberry root (dry or fresh), finely chopped
> Alcohol or vegetable glycerin

1. Prepare the blackberry root as a tincture, following the instructions on page 106.

2. To use, mix 1 teaspoon of the tincture in ½ cup warm water, juice, or herbal tea, and administer ¼ teaspoon of this preparation every hour.

Diarrhea Remedy Tea

To make this tea more palatable, you can add a small amount of maple syrup or blackberry juice concentrate (available in natural foods stores) for flavor.

> 3 parts blackberry root
> 2 parts marsh mallow root
> 1 part licorice root
> ⅛ part cinnamon bark

1. Mix the herbs and store in an airtight container until ready to use.

2. To use, prepare the herb mixture as a decoction, following the instructions on page 97. Administer according to the child's size and age, following the dosage guidelines beginning on page 91, and dosing the child every 30 to 45 minutes until symptoms subside.

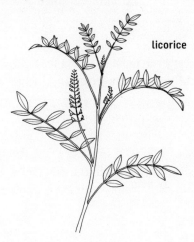

licorice

CONSTIPATION

CONSTIPATION IS OFTEN THE RESULT of eating foods that are "hot and dry" or difficult to digest, along with inadequate fluid intake. Constipation in children can also be a result of an unease or unwillingness in using the toilet. Children may be unwilling to use the bathroom because they are preoccupied with play or inattentive to the signals their body is giving them. Or they may be reluctant to use the bathroom because of a previous bad experience, or because they feel the bathroom does not offer privacy (as may be the case in a public setting, for example). Whatever the reason, if children do not permit themselves regular bowel movements, their stool hardens, resulting in constipation.

Be on the watch for such behaviors, assessing your child's toilet habits on a regular basis. Catching the problem early may eliminate a lifetime of stressful elimination.

Constipation can also result from a change in diet, certain medications, and excessive consumption of certain foods. High-fat dairy products, wheat, eggs, and refined, processed foods are generally the most common food culprits.

If your child develops constipation, the first step is to have him or her avoid foods that contribute to the problem, such as refined wheat products (like pasta, bread, and crackers) and hard cheeses; a nursing mother whose baby is experiencing constipation would do well to avoid these foods also. At the same time, it's helpful to add to the diet foods that contribute to healthy elimination: fruits, vegetables, whole grains, liquids, molasses, dried fruit (particularly apricots and prunes), and moist, cooling foods like oatmeal and Marsh Mallow Gruel (see page 42). A constipated child who is bottle-fed cow's milk might try switching to goat, rice, or soy milk.

Several herbs in particular can be helpful: carob powder, marsh mallow root or slippery elm bark, flaxseed, psyllium seed, licorice root, and Irish moss. These plants can be powdered and added to the child's meals. Give 1 to 4 teaspoons three or four times daily, or as often as needed during constipation. For children under the age of 10, use the smaller dose. These herbs are not laxative herbs per se but provide necessary bulk in the diet.

The following suggestions, combined with the dietary recommendations above, should bring relief to the child plagued by constipation:

- **Acidophilus and other probiotics.** Administer ½ teaspoon of acidophilus (use a product designed for children) with meals. Acidophilus adds friendly bacteria to the digestive tract and aids in good digestion
- **Bulk-building herbs.** Grind equal amounts of marsh mallow root (or slippery elm bark), flaxseed, and psyllium seed together until finely powdered. Mix ½ to 1 teaspoon of the mixture in with food at each meal. Carob, another herb that encourages smooth bowel movements, can also be added.
- **Bulk-building "candy."** Make a special bulk-building "candy" with dried fruits and powdered herbs. Grind prunes, figs, apricots, and raisins together. Mix in powdered psyllium seed, powdered marsh mallow root or slippery elm bark,

and fennel seed. Add enough carob powder to thicken. Roll into balls and serve daily as a delicious, nourishing snack. (See page 98 for more on candy balls.)

- **Triphala.** If constipation is persistent, give the child Triphala, an Ayurvedic formula made up of three medicinal fruits. Triphala is one of the most popular remedies for bowel irregularities and is used by thousands of people around the world. Though not a laxative, Triphala will help regulate digestion and stimulate sluggish bowels. Dosages on product packaging are generally designed for adults; see page 92 for dosage guidelines for children.

- **Water.** Be sure the child drinks plenty of room-temperature water. If morning constipation is the norm, give the child, upon rising, warm psyllium seed water (soak ½ teaspoon psyllium seed in ½ cup water overnight; add lemon juice and honey or maple syrup to taste). The child should drink ¼ to ½ cup, depending on his or her age and size.

- **Fresh and dried fruit.** Eating plenty of fruit can help regulate bowel movements. Fresh fruit is excellent. Also try soaking dried fruit, such as apricots and prunes, overnight and having your child eat them first thing in the morning. Organic is best. If the dried fruit is organic, encourage your child to drink the water that the fruit has soaked in, or use it in cooking cereal.

- **Exercise.** Exercise is critical for regular bowel movements. Getting enough exercise is generally not a problem for most children, but you may choose to make a regular time to do some activities together. A morning walk is a good way to get the energy moving and is also a nice opportunity to spend time together. The primary goal is to provide some centered, peaceful activity every day that gets the body moving vigorously while relaxing the mind and spirit.

Tea to Relieve Constipation

This blend stimulates sluggish bowels and encourages smooth bowel movements.

    4   parts fennel seed
    2   parts psyllium seed
    1   part licorice root
    1   part marsh mallow root
    ½   part cinnamon bark
         Pinch of stevia leaf to sweeten

1. Combine all the ingredients and store in an airtight container until ready to use.

2. To prepare, brew the herbs as a decoction, following the instructions on page 97. Strain.

3. Give ⅛–½ cup of the tea with meals, or as often as needed.

EARACHES

UNTIL A CHILD IS THREE OR FOUR years old, the ear canals are not fully formed and, consequently, do not drain well. When a child gets congested or has a cold, the ear canals often get plugged up with excess mucus, which then cannot drain properly. Bacteria begin to grow in the moisture of the accumulated secretions, and infection often occurs.

Ear infections can also result from allergies. If, despite your best efforts, your child has recurring ear infections, consider the possibility of allergies. Sugar, citrus, and dairy products, including milk, cheese, and ice cream, are the most common offenders. Wheat is also a big culprit, and many parents are finding that their children are healthier and have fewer allergies when wheat is removed from their diet.

Ear infections can be serious. Treated improperly, they can leave a child with hearing impairment. So it is important to treat an ear infection at its onset and to work in conjunction with a holistic health care practitioner and your family pediatrician. Watch for the early signs: congestion, runny nose, fever, and excessive rubbing or pulling of the ear lobe, combined with irritability and fussiness. If your child wakes up crying in the night and pulling at her ears, an infection has worked its way into the ear canals and will need to be attended to immediately.

Most pediatricians will prescribe antibiotics for an ear infection. But antibiotics, though sometimes effective for acute situations, do not correct the cause of the problem, and they can create havoc in a young child's system, disrupting the immune cycle and making the child further susceptible to disease. Also, as we're witnessing today, the overuse of antibiotics is causing a huge problem in our health care system and environment. Therefore, whenever you're using antibiotics, it is important to follow the suggestions outlined below, both to support the child's body in processing the antibiotics and to support the efficacy of those antibiotics.

Rest and Simple Remedies

It is imperative that a child with an ear infection get plenty of rest. He or she should not go out into the cold air prematurely. It is a common mistake to think a child has recovered from an ear infection and send him or her out to play too soon. So many times have I heard parents tell me, "Johnny kept me awake crying all night with a bad ear infection. Come morning he was fine, so I sent him off to school. But wouldn't you know it, that ear infection was back in full force again the next night." Ear infections have a way of doing that.

Seriously consider keeping a child with an ear infection housebound for at least a few days, until recovery is complete. Generally the reason we don't do this is because of the inconvenience it would cause in our insanely busy lives. Who really has the time or "luxury" these days to stay home to care for a sick child? However, keep in mind that the time spent caring for a sick child at the outset of illness often means far less time lost in the long run.

When a child has an ear infection, avoid giving him or her those foods that cause congestion and further exacerbate the condition. These foods include sugar and sugar-rich food, dairy products, especially milk and cheese, wheat products, orange juice (yes, orange juice), and most refined, processed foods.

Acidophilus and other probiotic cultures, given in doses of ½ teaspoon several times daily, can be very helpful for ear infections. Also try a tasty tea of fresh-grated ginger, fresh-squeezed lemon, and honey or maple syrup. It is a refreshing, decongesting blend.

Know the Cause of an Ear Infection

Please note that the garlic-mullein oil treatment on page 64 is only appropriate when the ear infection has been caused by congestion in the ear canals. When water is the culprit, adding oil can make the infection worse. Be sure you know whether the ear infection is caused by congestion or by water in the ear (swimmer's ear). How to tell the difference? If the ear pain is accompanied by a runny nose, cough, or other cold and flu symptoms, then most likely the infection is due to congestion. If there are no signs of congestion or cold or flu symptoms, and the child has recently been swimming or gotten water in his or her ear during a long bath or shower, then the infection is most likely caused by water in the ear.

If the infection is caused by water in the ear, do not treat with oil. Instead, use rubbing alcohol, witch hazel extract, apple cider vinegar, or St. John's wort tincture, which will help the water to

---

According to traditional Chinese medicine, the health of the kidneys is directly connected to the health of the ears; I've found this to be true as well. Note, however, that this treatment should be combined with other therapies for optimal results. To help support the kidneys, be certain the child is drinking sufficient fluids, like water; cranberry juice is a good choice, too, as it is a strengthening tonic for the kidneys. And try placing warm packs over the lower back (the area of the kidneys).

---

evaporate. You can add a drop of tea tree or lavender essential oil to the rubbing alcohol/vinegar/witch hazel or tincture to help fight the infection. Just drop a few drops of the preparation down each ear and massage it in. Placing a warm pack over the ear can be pain relieving and comforting at the same time.

If your child's ear infection isn't responding to your herbal home treatments in a day or two, if the pain and infection continue to get worse, or if pus or blood drains from the ear, then the eardrum may have ruptured, and you should seek medical help immediately. This sounds scary, I know. But use common sense. Most ear infections will heal up fine with simple home treatments and commonsense approaches. Eardrums seldom rupture when the infection is treated immediately, and if they do, unless the infection has been terribly neglected and/or repeats frequently, ruptured ears usually heal fine over time, with no hearing loss.

Garlic and Mullein Flower Oil

This is one of the best herbal remedies for ear infections caused by congestion. It is important to treat both ears; the ear canals are connected and the infection can move back and forth. Garlic has powerful antibiotic properties and is renowned for fighting infections. Mullein flower provides pain relief and also aids in fighting infections. St. John's wort is a strong antiviral and antibacterial agent and also has pain-relieving properties. With this combination of herbs, the oil not only helps fight the infection but also relieves the pain. Be absolutely sure the oil is warm, not hot.

> 2–3 tablespoons chopped garlic
>
> 2–3 tablespoons mullein flowers (fresh flowers are best, but dried flowers may be used)
>
> 2–3 tablespoons St. John's wort flowers (optional)
>
> Olive oil

1. Infuse the garlic, mullein, and St. John's wort (if using) in the olive oil, following the instructions on page 111.

2. To use, warm a teaspoon or so of the oil. Warm *only* to the temperature of mother's milk (about room temperature). Suction the oil into a dropper. Have the child lie down on his or her side, and drop several drops into the ear facing up. Wait for a minute or so, gently massaging the ear, and then have the child turn over so that you can drop several drops into the other ear. Any extra oil will drain out on its own within a few minutes.

3. Administer the warm herbal oil every 30 minutes, or as often as needed.

Ear Infection Formula

You can administer this formula as a tincture, as directed below. Or you can powder and encapsulate these herbs to administer to older children.

> 1 part echinacea root
> 1 part garlic (fresh)
> 1 part reishi mushroom (dried, cut, or powdered)
> ¼ part elderberry
> ¼ part goldenseal root (organically cultivated)
> Alcohol or vegetable glycerin

1. Prepare the herbs as a tincture, following the instructions on page 106.

2. To use, administer ⅛ teaspoon of the tincture diluted in warm water or juice orally three times daily.

FEVERS

A FEVER ITSELF IS A NATURAL mechanism to rid the body of infection and is a sign of a healthy immune system. It is only when the fever gets too high or lingers for too long that it can be debilitating, or even devastating. If your child's fever reaches 102°F/39°C or more, or lasts for several days, contact your holistic health care provider or pediatrician immediately. But otherwise, see fever as the useful tool it is. It is an important part of the immune system response.

Use the following techniques to help your child get through a fever and, when necessary, lower a fever.

Hydration

With small children, it is imperative to keep fluid intake high during a fever. Dehydration is the greatest danger of a childhood fever, not the actual temperature of the fever. So make sure any child with a fever is drinking adequate amounts of water, herbal tea, or diluted juice.

Children who are ill may not be eager to eat or drink anything. So how do we get adequate amounts of fluid into them? Give them a straw, as it makes drinking easier, especially from a prone position — a fancy straw will make it more fun! Make sure the liquid is at room temperature, as a high or low water temperature can interfere with absorption. Make sure the liquid is tasty, so the child wants to drink it; a little maple syrup or honey can be just the thing to make the drink inviting, adding a bit of nourishment as well.

Enemas are most helpful in hydrating a feverish child, especially when he or she won't or can't drink enough water; see page 110 for instructions. Enemas were once a common method for lowering fevers, but today people prefer to give children acetaminophen and other anti-inflammatory medicines that don't allow our natural-born immunity to step up and do the job. Of course, if the fever continues to rise and the child is getting worse, not better, then that's the time to reach for the medication. But doesn't it make more sense to use medicine that is supportive and works with our immune system, rather than suppressing it? Doesn't treating the underlying issues, rather than suppressing them, make for a healthier child in the long run?

Apple Cider Vinegar Treatments

To lower a fever, one old-fashioned and effective treatment is to bathe the child in a tepid or warm bath. Mix ¼ cup apple cider vinegar into the bathwater. Be certain there are no drafts in the room. After the bath, quickly wrap the child in a warm flannel sheet. Spritzing the sheet with a couple of drops of calming, soothing chamomile essential oil, diluted in a bit of water, can be very helpful.

Another fever-reducing treatment is to wrap the child's feet in a cool cloth that has been dipped in a mixture of apple cider vinegar and water. Keep the child bundled warmly.

Fever-Reducing Tea

This is a classic formula for treating colds, flus, and fevers. Variations of it can be found in health food stores and markets today.

> 2 parts catnip leaf
> 2 parts elder blossom
> 1 part echinacea root
> 1 part peppermint leaf

1. Mix the herbs and store in an airtight container until ready to use.

2. To prepare, pour 1 cup boiling water over 1 teaspoon of the mixture and let steep, covered, for 1 hour.

3. Administer every 30 minutes, following the dosage guidelines beginning on page 91.

CHICKEN POX, MEASLES, AND OTHER SKIN ERUPTIONS

CHICKEN POX AND MEASLES are a great discomfort, but most children sail through them with a little support and natural home treatments. Though they are distinctly different diseases, their treatment is similar.

When treating these common childhood illnesses, your aim should be to aid the body's natural defense mechanisms. The following treatments are geared toward supporting the body's immune reactions and its innate ability to respond to these disorders. However, be sure to involve your pediatrician if the child is under two years of age, and always be more cautious and vigilant with measles.

Super Immunity Syrup

This formula can also be made into a tea, but you'll need to add some pleasant-tasting herbs such as lemon balm and lemongrass for flavor. This immune-boosting syrup assists the body in warding off infection, supports the deep immune response, and lessens the uncomfortable effects of the rash.

> 2 parts elderberry
>
> 2 parts green milky oats
>
> 1 part astragalus root
>
> 1 part burdock root
>
> 1 part echinacea root and flowering top
>
> Honey or another sweetener of your choice

1. Prepare the herbs as a syrup, following the instructions on page 102 and sweetening with honey.

2. At the onset of infection, administer 1 teaspoon every hour until symptoms clear. Administer 4–6 times daily during the course of an infection.

Itch-Calming Tea

Children are itchy and irritable when they have chicken pox, measles, and other skin irritations. This nervine tea will help soothe both conditions — the itchiness and the irritation.

> 2 parts lemon balm leaf
> 2 parts green milky oats
> 1 part calendula flower
> 1 part passionflower
> 1 part red clover blossom
> Stevia leaf, honey, or maple syrup to sweeten

1. Mix the herbs and store in an airtight container until ready to use.

2. To prepare, pour 1 cup boiling water over 1 teaspoon of the herb mixture and let steep, covered, for 30 minutes. Strain, and sweeten to taste with stevia, honey, or maple syrup.

3. Let the child drink as much as desired.

Valerian-Burdock Tincture
for Itching and Skin Rash

This is my favorite formula to help relieve itching and promote relaxation. You can also purchase burdock root, echinacea, and valerian tinctures ready-made from most natural foods stores; mix them together in the proportions given below.

2 parts burdock root

1 part echinacea root

1 part valerian root

   Alcohol or vegetable glycerin

1. Prepare the herbs as a tincture, following the instructions on page 106.

2. To use, administer ⅛ teaspoon of the tincture diluted in warm water or juice three times daily.

Note: For some children, valerian acts as a stimulant. If you notice your child becoming more irritated and active after using this tincture, discontinue use.

Oatmeal Bath

Nothing is as soothing to itchy, irritated skin as a warm oatmeal bath. For extra comfort, place the strained oatmeal in a cotton bag or sock and add it to the bathwater. Consider adding a few drops of lavender essential oil, which, in addition to being a relaxing nervine that will help with the irritation and itching, has antibacterial and disinfectant properties.

          2 cups oats
      8–10 cups water
            Lavender essential oil (optional)

1. Combine the oats with the water in a big pot. Bring to a boil, and let simmer for 5 minutes. Then strain, reserving the liquid (and the oats, if you like).

2. Pour the liquid into a full tub of water. Add a drop or two of lavender essential oil, if desired. Have your child bathe for as long as he or she likes — and as often as he or she likes — in the warm, soothing water.

Disinfectant Powder

Mix up this herbal powder and keep on hand as a disinfectant. It can be sprinkled directly on oozing pox sores, helping to dry them as well as preventing infection from setting in. You may also try sprinkling slippery elm powder over the sores. It's so soothing and helps stop the itching, but it won't have the same disinfectant properties as this powder.

          1 ounce green clay (available from natural food and herb stores)
          1 tablespoon calendula flower powder
          1 tablespoon comfrey root powder
          ½ tablespoon goldenseal root powder (organically cultivated)

1. Combine all the ingredients. Store in a shaker container or glass bottle with a tight-fitting lid.

2. Sprinkle as needed on skin sores to stop itching and promote drying.

COLDS AND FLUS

THERE'S PROBABLY NOT a person alive who escaped childhood without at least a cold or two. Unless these all-too-common maladies are recurrent, there's no need for concern. The various "bugs" that cause colds and flus allow the immune system to kick into action, "schooling" it to do its job better and more efficiently. Colds also provide the opportunity for us to observe how quickly our bodies respond to common illnesses, and our immune response to them serves as an indicator of our overall health and resiliency.

Grandma knew best! Lots of fluids, warm soup, a couple days of rest, and some immune-strengthening herbs — that's generally all that's needed. If your child suffers from recurrent colds or is having difficulty recovering from a particularly devastating flu, then seek the guidance of a holistic health care provider or your family doctor.

Vitamin C Therapy

Another tactic I've found helpful in fighting colds and flus is to give high doses (up to 5,000 milligrams) of vitamin C, usually in liquid form. Start with a smaller dose, and increase gradually. If the child develops runny stools, decrease the amount. High doses of vitamin C do seem to help kick the immune response into action. It works best at the onset of colds and flus, helping to prevent or lessen the symptoms.

At the first sign of a cold or flu, start giving your child frequent, higher-than-normal doses of echinacea tincture, which will jump-start the immune system. For example, a child of four would take ⅛ teaspoon of echinacea tincture every hour until the symptoms subside. I like to mix echinacea tincture with equal parts of elderberry syrup (see the recipe on the next page). You can put this mixture in a spritzer bottle and spray directly in the mouth, minding the guidelines for appropriate dosages (see pages 91–93).

Super Immunity Tincture

Though echinacea is often effective by itself, a stronger immune support tincture may be used instead of or in addition to the echinacea. Though not as well known in the United States, spilanthes has properties similar to those of echinacea, but with even stronger antiviral and antimicrobial properties. Here is one of my favorite formulas that uses both echinacea and spilanthes.

> 2 parts echinacea root, leaf, and flower
> 2 parts licorice root
> 1 part spilanthes flower and leaf
> ½ part garlic
> ½ part dried reishi mushroom
> Alcohol or vegetable glycerin

1. Prepare the herbs and mushroom as a tincture, following the instructions on page 106.

2. To use, follow the dosage guidelines beginning on page 91. This tincture will not taste good, so dilute the dosage in a bit of juice or herb tea to help disguise the flavor.

Elderberry Syrup

This is the most popular herbal cold and flu remedy in Europe, and it's delicious. Every year I try to make two or three batches of elderberry syrup, and it's always gone by the end of the season. I've gathered fresh elderberries from the West Coast to the East Coast and have marked the seasons by the ripening of these dark blue-black berries. Use only blue elderberries; the red ones are potentially toxic if eaten in large quantities.

> 2 cups fresh or 1 cup dried elderberries
> 3–4 cups water
> 1–2 cups honey or another sweetener of your choice

1. Place the berries in a saucepan and cover with the water. Simmer over low heat for 30–45 minutes. Smash the berries in the pan, then strain the mixture through a fine-mesh strainer. Sweeten to taste with the honey. Store in the refrigerator, where the syrup will keep for 2–3 months.

2. To use, follow the dosage guidelines beginning on page 91.

Ginger-Echinacea Syrup

This truly delicious syrup is very effective for treating "wet," hacking coughs and colds that have moved into the lungs. Other herbs can be added as desired, such as wild cherry bark and licorice root for a cough, elecampane for respiratory infection, or valerian for spastic coughing, anxiety, and restlessness.

> 1 part dried echinacea root
> 1 part fresh ginger root
> Honey or another sweetener of your choice

1. Prepare the herbs as a syrup, following the instructions on page 101 and sweetening with honey.

2. To use, follow the dosage guidelines beginning on page 91. Ginger is very warming; if the syrup is too "hot" for your child's taste, serve the syrup diluted in warm water or tea.

Cough Be Gone & Sore Throat Syrup

For a sore throat and irritated, dry cough, this soothing tasty syrup is just the remedy. If the cough is spastic and/or continuous, add more valerian to the formula. Valerian is an antispasmodic and helps relax muscles throughout the body.

>   4 parts fennel seed
>   2 parts licorice root
>   2 parts slippery elm bark (ethically harvested)
>   2 parts wild cherry bark
>   1–2 parts valerian root
>   1 part cinnamon bark
>   ½ part ginger root
>   ⅛ part orange peel
>   Honey or another sweetener of your choice

1. Prepare the herbs as a syrup, following the instructions on page 101 and sweetening with honey.

2. To use, follow the dosage guidelines beginning on page 91.

Feed a Cold?

What and how much a sick child eats will greatly affect the degree of his or her illness. All dairy products, especially milk and ice cream, tend to make the symptoms of a cold worse. I'm aware of how easy this is to say, and how difficult it is to say no to a child, especially a child who is ill. However, to the extent that you can convince your child to eat healthy, immune-supportive foods and avoid those foods that agitate the illness, you'll help your child recover more quickly. All sugar-rich foods should be avoided. So should orange juice, in spite of what the glossy ads say. A large, ice-cold glass of orange juice, no matter how good it tastes, is very acidic and will create more mucus and congestion. Instead, try hot lemonade made with fresh-squeezed lemon juice, a pinch of ginger, and a little honey or maple syrup to sweeten. Lemons provide vitamin C, are alkalizing, and will help prevent illness.

Grandma's chicken soup (or, if you're a vegetarian, miso or vegetable broth) is really the best thing to eat when you have a cold or flu. The mineral-rich broth, the fluid, and the warmth are all beneficial. I often add medicinal herbs directly to the soup base. Astragalus, dandelion root, burdock root, and echinacea root, for example, can be cooked in the broth for extra immune support, nourishment, and vitality. Steamed grains, such as millet and quinoa, are better than pasta when a child is ill. Hot oatmeal is going to be much better than cold cereal, especially cold cereal served with milk. In fact, hot oatmeal is generally going to be better than most cold cereals even when your child is well. When you put on your reading glasses and examine the fine print on cereal boxes, it's a bit shocking to see what we're feeding our children.

Treating a Runny Nose and Sinus Congestion

An instant remedy for sinus congestion and a runny nose is an herbal steam. Heat a large pot of water until steaming, and add a drop or two of eucalyptus essential oil and/or a handful of fresh eucalyptus leaves (thyme and rosemary will work also). Set the pot on a low table, and have the child lean over it to inhale this steam. Cover the child's head and the pot with a large towel to capture the steam. Treat for 5 to 10 minutes, or until the sinuses open up. Instruct the child to keep his or her eyes closed, as the herbal oils can make them tear up and cause some discomfort. And, of course, make sure your child doesn't touch the very hot pot (or pour the steaming water into a heat-resistant bowl). Do not use the steam for children under four years old. This treatment is even better if you spend a few minutes massaging your child's shoulders and back while he or she is steaming. Your healing touch may be just the thing that heals.

Treating Lung and Chest Congestion

A hot water bottle placed on the back, between the shoulder blades, helps loosen up phlegm and deep-seated congestion in the chest. I use an old-fashioned hot water bottle wrapped in cotton flannel to keep in the heat. It's even more effective if you first rub Bag Balm, Tiger Balm, Vicks VapoRub, or a homemade vapor-type salve over the child's back and chest. Because the oils can be irritating, especially to the eyes, don't let the child apply these salves on him- or herself. Do it yourself — and be careful not to put too much on that tender young skin.

The technique called "hand cupping" — in layman's terms, thumping on the upper back — can help loosen phlegm and congestion. Curve the palm of your hand inward to make a cup (like you would if you were drinking water from your hands), and use it to gently thump the child's upper back. It feels good and really helps loosen phlegm from deep in the lungs. If needed, follow with a good cup of tea that helps expel mucus (see the recipe below).

Lung & Chest Congestion Formula

This formula can be made into a tea, syrup, or tincture and is very effective in clearing up bronchial congestion. If making a tea, adjust the flavors by adding more licorice, cinnamon, and ginger to the formula.

> 2 parts licorice root
> 1 part cinnamon bark
> 1 part echinacea root
> 1 part elecampane root
> ¼ part ginger root and/or cinnamon bark

1. Combine the ingredients and store in an airtight container until ready to use.

2. To make tea, prepare as a decoction, following the instructions on page 97. To make tincture, see page 106 for instructions. To make a syrup, see page 101. Administer according to the child's size and age, following the guidelines beginning on page 91.

BURNS, CUTS, SCRAPES, AND INSECT BITES

INVARIABLY, ALL CHILDREN GET burns, cuts, scrapes, bee stings, and bug bites. These are perfect opportunities to teach them the art of self-care and make them "little healers." When you're making herbal salves and homemade remedies for your first-aid cabinet, include your children in the process. Most children love to participate in these activities and are much keener to use a medicine they've made themselves. What's even more fun is to go out with them to pick the common garden "weeds" that are powerful healing plants. Plantain, dandelion, burdock, chickweed — all grow in abundance around us, even in cities. Teach your children early to appreciate these healing gifts and how to use them in healing salves and teas.

Treating Burns

Salve. The all-purpose salve on page 52 is excellent for first- and even second-degree burns. I'm not even sure where the recipe originated, but it's been circulating for as long as I've been practicing herbalism. It's a must-have remedy in every household with small children.

Honey. Another remedy that I have used on both minor and severe (second-degree) burns is a mixture of 1 tablespoon honey with 1 or 2 drops peppermint essential oil. Honey has been used for centuries as an antiseptic dressing for burns. The addition of the peppermint essential oil helps "cool" the burn. On a minor burn, it will relieve pain almost instantly. The honey also keeps the burn clean and free from infection.

Lavender. Lavender essential oil is another gentle, safe healing agent for burns and is both soothing and disinfectant.

Aloe. The fresh gel from the aloe vera plant is also tremendously cooling and healing for burns. Choose a large, succulent leaf and slice it carefully off the mother plant. The plant will ooze a gel-like substance and heal itself where you've cut it. Slice along the edge of the leaf lengthwise (cutting only as far as you need to for one application of gel). Scoop out the gel from the inside of the leaf, scraping the skin clean. This gel can be applied directly to any burn, as well as other kinds of wounds and rashes. (But note: Never use aloe vera gel on a staph infection. It will seal in the bacteria, creating a perfect petri environment for the staph to multiply. If you suspect staph, it's best not to use aloe vera.)

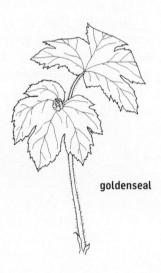

goldenseal

Healing Clay

Clay is composed of mineral-rich deposits accumulated over millions of years. Green clay is particularly rich in minerals and is the one I prefer to use in first-aid remedies. You can buy green clay in most natural foods or herb stores, and it is a wonderful healing agent when used alone or in combination with herbs for cuts, wounds, and insect bites. To treat burns or hot, itchy rashes, add a few drops of peppermint essential oil to the clay paste before you apply it; peppermint oil is cooling and soothing.

 4 parts clay
 1 part comfrey root powder
 1 part aloe vera powder
 1 part goldenseal root (organically cultivated) or chaparral
    powder

1. Mix the clay with the powdered herbs. Store in a glass jar.

2. To use, mix a small amount of the clay mixture with enough water to form a paste and apply directly to cuts, wounds, and insect bites.

Alternatively, you can premix the clay and herbal powders into a paste with water. Add a few drops of lavender and tea tree essential oils, which offer both antiseptic and preservative properties. Store the clay paste in a glass jar with a tight-fitting lid. If the paste dries out, just remoisten with water.

TONIC TEAS FOR GOOD HEALTH

INCLUDED HERE ARE SOME OF MY FAVORITE tea recipes for promoting good health in children. Each of the teas tastes delicious and can be drunk either by itself or mixed with fruit juice to sweeten. If there is a particular tea recipe your child most enjoys or needs, I suggest mixing up a quart of the blend to keep on hand. Stored in the refrigerator, it will last several days.

To encourage your children to become involved in their own self-care (and to have greater interest in actually drinking the teas), have them get involved in making these tea blends. Let your children name their remedies and make labels for them. These tea blends make wonderful, original gifts to give to other children that will stand out amidst the manufactured plastic toys of today. You can include a special cup and even a teapot. When my granddaughter Lily was just a few years old, I gave her a tea set, and she treasures it. Every year I mix up and give her some of her own special tea blends.

Calming Tonic Tea

This blend is especially useful for calming a fussy child. It is gently soothing and can be used over an extended period of time as a tonic for the nervous system. This blend is also helpful during stressful situations such as colic, fever, and teething.

> 2 parts chamomile flower
> 2 parts lemon balm leaf
> 2 parts green milky oats
> 1 part catnip leaf

1 part rose petals
1 part hawthorn berries, flowers, and/or leaves
   Pinch of stevia leaf to sweeten

1. Combine all the ingredients and store in an airtight container until ready to use.

2. To prepare, brew as an infusion, following the instructions on page 96. This is a tonic, so your child can drink as much of it as he or she wants.

High C Tea

This wonderfully refreshing blend provides bioflavonoids and vitamin C in an organic, naturally biochelated base so that all the nutrients are readily available for absorption. The high level of vitamins found in commercial vitamins are therapeutic dosages, and they may be useful to combat illness, but for daily maintenance this tea, with its natural dose, is better for your child.

4 parts rose hips
3 parts hibiscus flower
2 parts lemongrass
1 part spearmint leaf
⅛ part orange peel and/or cinnamon chips
   Pinch of stevia leaf to sweeten

1. Combine all the ingredients and store in an airtight container until ready to use.

2. To prepare, brew as an infusion, following the instructions on page 96. This is a tonic, so your child can drink as much of it as he or she wants.

Respiratory Tonic Tea

This blend is an effective and tasty tea for building strong, healthy lungs. It is especially helpful for children who have recurring respiratory problems such as colds, flu, hay fever, asthma, ear infections, and general congestion. This tea is not necessarily the blend you might choose to use in the acute stages of a respiratory infection, but when used over a period of time, it will aid in establishing a healthy respiratory system.

> 2 parts fennel seed
> 2 parts red clover blossom
> 2 parts rose hips
> 2 parts lemongrass
> 1 part calendula flower
> 1 part coltsfoot leaf
> 1 part mullein leaf

1. Combine all the ingredients and store in an airtight container until ready to use.

2. To prepare, brew as an infusion, following the instructions on page 96. Administer according to the child's size and age, following the dosage guidelines beginning on page 91.

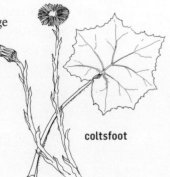

coltsfoot

RECIPES FOR BABY-CARE PRODUCTS

THOUGH THERE IS A WONDERFUL VARIETY of natural baby-care products on the market these days, it's delightful, simple, and far less costly to make your own. When I first started making my own baby products, I was a young, single, working mom. Cost was certainly a factor for me, but not nearly as important as the purity of the product. The only baby products available at the time were the typical commercial ones, and they were far from natural. So I decided to make my own. Forty-five years later, these products are still popular and have been used by hundreds of parents and their children. All are 100 percent natural and are easy and fun to make — and it's always fun to adjust the formulas, adding your own favorite ingredients to make your own unique creations.

Baby's Bath Herbs

Use the following mixture in the bath. These herbs are soothing and relaxing — for Mom and Dad, too.

> 2 parts calendula flower
> 2 parts chamomile flower
> 1 part lavender flower
> 1 part rose petals

1. Combine all the herbs and store in an airtight container until ready to use.

2. To use, prepare the blend as an herbal bath, following the instructions on page 103.

Baby's Sweet Sleep Pillow

Create a very special pillow to soothe your infant into a peaceful sleep with the calming, soothing, aromatic herbs in this blend. Herbal sleep pillows have proven helpful for many children who have trouble sleeping. I think every child should have one.

        2   parts chamomile flower
        1   part hops strobile
        1   part lavender flower
        1   part rose petals
    1–2   drops lavender essential oil (optional)
        1   (6- by 6-inch) piece soft fabric (flannel is wonderful)

1. Combine the herbs in a bowl. Add a drop or two of lavender essential oil and mix well.

2. Stitch three sides of a 6- by 6-inch cotton "pillow," leaving one end open for stuffing. Fill abundantly with the herb mixture. Place near your baby's head to help promote peaceful, aromatic sleep.

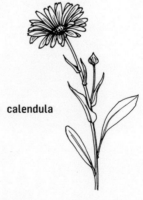

calendula

Baby's Blessed Bath & Bottom Oil

This is excellent all-purpose oil, useful for not only preventing diaper rash but also as a massage oil. Try giving your child a gentle massage after a bath. Teach your child early the art and value of touch. So often these days people feel disconnected and lonely because they simply forget to touch one another. After you massage your child's sweet little body, teach him or her to massage your own hands or back, so the child, too, is learning the healing art of touching and massage . . . and the equally fine art of giving and receiving.

2 parts calendula flower
1 part chamomile flower
1 part comfrey leaf
1 part rose petals
   Apricot kernel, almond, olive oil, or a combination of these

1. Infuse the herbs in the oil, following the instructions on page 111.

2. To use, massage the oil on your baby's skin after baths, and on your baby's bottom as a preventive at the first sign of diaper rash.

CHAPTER FOUR

HOW TO MAKE HERBAL REMEDIES

How do you make herbal remedies for children? And, how do you make them not only effective but also tasty enough that even a picky child is willing to try them? This chapter will introduce you to the joyful and ancient art of herbal preparation, with an emphasis on remedies for children. Of course, not everyone enjoys "playing" in the kitchen. If making herbal remedies is not your cup of tea, don't despair. You can easily find high-quality herbal products in many natural food stores and herb shops, and also online. (For suggested companies, see the resources at the end of this book.)

Most often, making herbal remedies for children allows us the opportunity — or challenge, depending how you choose to embrace it — to be creative and innovative. The flavors of medicinal herbs are unfamiliar, and sometimes bitter, pungent, or sour, and children are often unwilling to try them. After all, when a child is sick, she sometimes is unwilling to eat even her favorite foods. Since consistency, when treating both adults and children, is the key to any herb's effectiveness, it is important to develop remedies that are pleasant and easy to take.

In the following pages you'll find some of my favorite ways to administer herbs to children. These suggestions come from years of observing what children will and will not accept. Each child, of course, is unique, and what is acceptable for one may not work for another. Each age group brings with it a different set of challenges. Be innovative and willing to work with the individual nature of each child.

Fresh or Dried Herbs?

Some herbs are better fresh, and others dried, and when it's necessary to use one or the other, the recipe will specify. Otherwise, whether you use fresh or dried herbs will depend on what's available and what type of remedy you're making. When possible, use fresh herbs to make teas and for cooking. Dried herbs are often better for making oils and salves because they have less water content (the water can encourage spoilage).

BUYING QUALITY HERBS

PURCHASE HIGH-QUALITY ORGANIC HERBS whenever possible. Though these herbs may cost a few cents more, they are far better for our children and our planet. Of course, it's even better if you can grow your own. To grow a little herb garden, you needn't have even one green thumb, but just a little plot of soil, sunshine, water, and a bit of time. And it's a perfect activity to share with young children and another away to ensure they get their hands in the dirt to connect with nature.

Don't use herbs that are endangered or at risk. Part of our responsibility in using herbs today is to preserve not only the ancient traditions of herbalism but also the plants the traditions are based on. To learn more about endangered herbs, contact the United Plant Savers (see resources on page 119).

STORAGE

HERBS RETAIN THEIR PROPERTIES BEST if stored in airtight glass jars, out of direct light, in a cool area. If you have small children in your household, store herbs in glass bottles with tight-fitting lids. Be sure to label the jars, for it becomes an impossible task to remember what's what in those little glass bottles. Store all herbs and remedies out of reach of children. One of the problems with many remedies for children is that they are made to taste appealing. Thankfully, most of your herbal remedies won't be harmful if ingested in larger amounts than intended. Still, keeping remedies out of reach and in well-sealed containers is a good general rule when there are small children about.

DETERMINING DOSAGE

THERE ARE SEVERAL DIFFERENT TECHNIQUES used to determine the proper dosage for children. Like parents who have grown accustomed to the needs of their children, most herbalists rely on years of experience and intuition to determine the safest and most effective dosage. If you are just beginning to use herbs and/or if you are using herbs you are unfamiliar with, then the following charts will prove helpful. They provide sound guidelines for prescribing the proper amount of herbs for children. But they are just guidelines, and it is equally important to consider the weight, height, and age of your child. Also consider the child's overall constitution: Is he or she generally

....

Determining a Child's Dosage by Young's and Cowling's Rules

These rules for dosage determination rely on mathematical calculations using the child's age.

Young's Rule: Add 12 to the child's age, and divide the child's age by this total. For example, let's say you are working with a four-year-old: 4 + 12 = 16. Then, 4 ÷ 16 = 0.25. So this child's dosage would be one-quarter of the adult dosage.

Cowling's Rule: Divide the child's age at his or her next birthday by 24. For example, let's say you are working with a child who is currently three years old. At his next birthday he'll turn four. So, 4 ÷ 24 = 0.16. So this child's dosage will be one-sixth of the adult dosage.

....

strong and healthy or sensitive and prone to illness? What is the nature of the illness and the quality and strength of the herbs being used? Balance these considerations with sound information and a healthy dash of common sense.

When the adult dosage is 1 cup (8 ounces)

AGE	DOSAGE
younger than 2 years	½ to 1 teaspoon
2 to 4 years	2 teaspoons
4 to 7 years	1 tablespoon
7 to 11 years	2 tablespoons

When the adult dosage is 1 teaspoon (60 drops)

AGE	DOSAGE
younger than 3 months	2 drops
3 to 6 months	3 drops
6 to 9 months	4 drops
9 to 12 months	5 drops
12 to 18 months	7 drops
18 to 24 months	8 drops
2 to 3 years	10 drops
3 to 4 years	12 drops
4 to 6 years	15 drops
6 to 9 years	24 drops
9 to 12 years	30 drops

Of course, to apply those dosage equivalents, you'll need to know the recommended dosage for adults. So the following chart gives basic guidelines for determining dosages for adults, based on whether the condition is chronic or acute.

Dosage Chart for Adults

Chronic problems are long-term imbalances such as asthma, poor immune function, and allergies. They usually develop slowly over a period of weeks or months and generally require a long-term commitment to correct the imbalance. Chronic problems can flare up and manifest acute symptoms, but the underlying problem is long-standing.

Acute problems come on suddenly, reach a crisis quickly, and need immediate response. Examples of acute problems include tooth-aches, earache, headaches, and burns. Pain is often an acute symptom, though it can be caused by either an acute or a chronic problem.

PREPARATION	DOSAGE FOR CHRONIC CONDITIONS	DOSAGE FOR ACUTE CONDITIONS
Tea	3–4 cups daily for 5 days, rest for 2 days, then repeat for several weeks, or until the problem is corrected	¼–½ cup throughout the day, up to 3–4 cups, until symptoms subside
Tinctures and syrups	½–1 teaspoon 3 times daily for 5 days, rest for 2 days, then continue for several weeks, or until the problem is corrected	¼–½ teaspoon every 30–60 minutes until symptoms subside
Capsules or tablets	2 capsules/tablets 3 times daily for 5 days, rest for 2 days, then continue for several weeks, or until the problem is corrected	1 capsule/tablet every hour until symptoms subside

HOW TO DETERMINE MEASUREMENTS

WHILE MANY PEOPLE ARE CONVERTING to the metric system, I've reverted to the simpler's method of measuring. Many herbalists choose to use this system because it is effective, simple, and versatile. Throughout this book measurements are referred to as "parts": 3 parts chamomile, 2 parts green milky oats, 1 part lemon balm. A "part" is any unit of measurement you want it to be: cups, ounces, pounds, tablespoons, or teaspoons. You'll use the same unit of measurement for each "part" in a recipe. The "part" measurement determines the ratio of ingredients in a recipe, and it allows you to make each recipe in the amount you need.

Sample Formula Blended in the Simpler's Method

PARTS	PARTS IN TABLESPOONS	PARTS IN TEASPOONS
3 parts chamomile	3 tablespoons chamomile	3 teaspoons chamomile
2 parts green milky oats	2 tablespoons green milky oats	2 teaspoons green milky oats
1 part lemon balm	1 tablespoon lemon balm	1 teaspoon lemon balm

While the simpler's method may not always be exact, it is exacting enough to make excellent herbal products. And remember, because you're using only gentle, safe herbs, and not any with the potential for toxicity, you don't need to be exact with your measurements. I often use the "pinch of this and dab of that" method of measuring with great success.

HERBAL TEAS

THE MAKING OF HERBAL TEA is a fine art, but it is also bless-edly simple. There are books written on the subject: how to choose the right accoutrements, the proper invitation to send, how warm to serve the chosen blend. I, too, have filled many pages with the art of making and serving herbal tea. But for simplicity's sake, all you really need is a quart jar with a tight-fitting lid, herbs, and water.

For a medicinal tea to be effective, it must be administered in small amounts several times daily. For chronic problems such as allergies, long-term respiratory issues, or nervous tension, serve the tea three to four times daily. For acute ailments such as colds, fevers, and headache, have the child take several small sips every half hour until the symptoms subside. Follow the dosage guidelines beginning on page 91.

To make a medicinal tea, use 1 to 3 tablespoons of herb for each cup of water. The herb-to-water ratio varies with the quality of herbs being used, whether the herb is fresh or dried (fresh herbs are used in greater amounts than dried), and how strong you wish the tea to be. With young children, start with the lesser amount. There are several methods of brewing.

Infusions

Infusions are teas made from the more delicate parts of the plant, including the leaves and flowers. Place the herb in a container, pour boiling water over it, and cover tightly. Let steep for 30 to 45 minutes. A tea intended only as refreshment would steep for much less time, but for medicinal purposes you want a more concentrated tea. The length of time you steep and the amount of herb you use will determine the strength (and flavor) of the tea.

....

Natural Sweeteners

There are many delicious and naturally sweet herbs that can be used to flavor the bitter and less palatable flavors of some medicinal herbs. Try sweetening your herbal teas with any of the following:

- Anise seed
- Chinese star anise
- Fennel seed
- Licorice root
- Marsh mallow root
- Stevia leaf
- Maple syrup, rice syrup, or honey

You can also make teas more tasty by adding familiar warming flavors, such as cinnamon, ginger, hibiscus, or mint. Or try mixing them with fruit juice. Warm apple juice is a favorite mixer, especially when paired with a cinnamon stick for added flavor. This often makes even the most bitter teas quite tasty and acceptable to young and old alike.

....

Decoctions

Decoctions are teas made from the more tenacious parts of the plant, such as the roots and bark. It's a little harder to extract the active constituents from these more woody parts, so a slow simmer (or an overnight infusion) is often required. Place the herb in a small saucepan and add cold water. Cover, bring to a slow simmer, and let simmer for approximately 20 minutes. Again, the length of time you simmer and the amount of herb you use will have a direct effect on the strength of the tea.

Solar and Lunar Infusions

Solar and lunar infusions utilize the light of the sun and moon to extract the healing properties of the herbs. What could be more fun, magical, and childlike? I believe we are children of the sky as well as the earth, and using these energies in our healing work adds a special touch. If nothing else, it's delightfully fun and adds a hint of magic and mystery to our kitchen work.

- **To make solar tea,** place 1 to 2 ounces of herb in 1 quart of water in a large jar. Put on the lid, place the jar in a spot that gets direct sunlight, and leave exposed to the sun for several hours.

- **To make lunar tea,** place 1 to 2 ounces of herb in 1 quart of water in a large jar or glass bowl. Place directly in the path of the moonlight. It's not necessary to place a lid on the container, unless there are a lot of night-flying bugs around. Leave overnight, then strain and drink first thing in the morning. Lunar tea is subtle and magical; it is whispered that fairies love to drink it!

MEDICINAL "CANDY" BALLS

ONE OF MY FAVORITE WAYS to give medicinal herbs to children is these "candy" balls. They are tasty and nutritious, as well as fun to make. This simple recipe calls for powdered herbs mixed into a paste with nut or seed butter, honey or some other sweetener, and/or ground-up dried fruits, but there are countless variations. Invite your children to help you make the candy. They are generally much more willing to take their daily "medicine" when it tastes good and they've had a hand in making it. Just be sure to keep it out of their reach once it's finished, or you may find that it's gone quicker than you wanted it to be!

Herbs must be finely powdered when used in these herbal candies. Though you can use home grinders, such as coffee grinders, to powder herbs, they aren't very efficient and don't generally powder the herbs finely enough. I've found it simpler and more efficient to purchase herbs in powdered form.

To determine the dosage, figure out how much of the herbal remedy you wish to give your child daily (see the discussion on page 91). Measure and add the appropriate amount of herb powders you mix into the candy "dough," and divide the dough into the appropriate number of balls. For instance, if you were giving ¼ teaspoon of the herb daily to your child, and you added 2 teaspoons total of herb powder into the candy dough, you would roll eight balls — each ball is a single daily dose containing ¼ teaspoon of the herb. Usually, I work with larger amounts, mixing in 1 to 2 ounces of herbal powders to yield a month's supply.

HOW TO MAKE CANDY BALLS WITH A NUT OR SEED BUTTER BASE

There are, of course, many variations of this recipe. Experiment and use the nut butters, seed butters, and sweeteners your child enjoys best. I myself prefer using a combination of butters, such as equal parts of almond butter and sesame seed butter (tahini). You'll need the following:

- 1 cup nut and/or seed butter (almond butter, peanut butter, cashew butter, tahini, sunflower seed butter)
- ¼–½ cup sweetener (honey, maple syrup, rice syrup)
- Finely powdered herb formula (amount determined by appropriate dosage)
- ¼ cup "goodies" (shredded coconut, chopped nuts, carob or chocolate chips, granola, raisins, cranberries, and so on)
- Carob powder or unsweetened cocoa powder
- Coconut flakes (optional)

Step 1. Combine the nut or seed butters with the sweetener, mixing well.

Step 2. Add the powdered herbs, and mix well.

Step 3. Stir in the goodies, followed by enough powdered carob or unsweetened cocoa powder to thicken the dough to the point that you can roll it into balls.

(continued on next page)

Step 4. Divide the dough into a number of portions such that each ball contains a single dose of the herb powders. Roll each piece into a ball. If you like, you can roll the balls in coconut flakes, carob powder, or cocoa powder; a simple way to do this is to place the coconut, carob, or cocoa in a small bag and shake the balls, one by one, in with the bag.

Step 5. Wrap the balls in wax paper and store in a cool place (the refrigerator is best for balls with nut butter, as they go rancid quickly).

HOW TO MAKE CANDY BALLS WITH A DRIED FRUIT BASE

A variation on the above recipe and another tasty way to get herbs into children is to make candy balls with a "dough" made from ground-up fruit and/or nuts. Dried fruits such as apricots, figs, apples, and dates, and nuts such as walnuts, almonds, hazel, and Brazil nuts are all great to use. Choose what your child enjoys most and what is best for their health. There are endless varieties to this basic recipe. Begin with the following:

- Dried fruits and nuts (the exact proportions are up to you)
- Finely powdered herb formula (amount determined by appropriate dosage)
- Coconut flakes, carob powder, or unsweetened cocoa powder

Step 1. Grind the dried fruits and nuts in a food processor or old-fashioned hand grinder. Mix well.

Step 2. Add the powdered herbs, and mix well.

Step 3. Add enough coconut flakes, carob powder, and/or unsweetened cocoa powder to thicken the dough to the point that you can roll it into balls.

Step 4. Divide the dough into a number of portions such that each ball contains a single dose of the herb powders. Roll each piece into a ball. Roll the balls in coconut flakes, carob powder, or cocoa powder.

Alternatively, you can flatten the dough in a pan and cut it into squares.

Step 5. Wrap the balls in wax paper and store in a cool place or the refrigerator.

SYRUPS

BECAUSE SYRUPS ARE SWEET, children often are very compliant when it comes to taking their herbal medicine in this form. (So are elderly people and everyone in between!) Syrups are delicious, concentrated extracts of herbs that are cooked slowly with a sweetener to create a thick, sweet liquid medicine. Though cooking may destroy some of an herb's healing constituents, syrups remain, nevertheless, an effective medicine, not least because children are so much more willing to take them than a tincture or capsule.

While we often think of syrups for coughs, colds, and flus, they are really quite appropriate for any number of illnesses. Almost any herbal formula can be made into syrup. If you prefer not to use honey in a syrup for younger children (because of fears of botulism), then substitute organic sugar, maple syrup (rich in minerals), and/or rice syrup.

HOW TO MAKE SYRUP

Step 1. Combine the herbs with water in a saucepan, using 2 to 3 ounces of herbs per quart of water. Over low heat, simmer the liquid down to 1 pint. This will give you a very concentrated, thick tea.

Step 2. Strain the herbs from the liquid. Any large strainer will do, but I've found a double-mesh stainless-steel strainer to work best. Compost the herbs and pour the liquid back into the pot.

Step 3. To each pint of liquid, add 1 to 2 cups of honey or other sweetener. Most recipes call for 2 cups of sweetener (a 1:1 ratio of sweetener to liquid), which I find far too sweet for my taste, but the added sugar helped preserve the syrup in the days when refrigeration wasn't common.

Step 4. Warm the honey and liquid together only enough to mix well. Most recipes instruct you to cook the syrup for 20 to 30 minutes longer over high heat to thicken it. It does certainly make thicker syrup, but I'd rather not cook the living enzymes out of the honey. Again, however, there are no hard and fast rules, just preferred methods of doing things.

Step 5. Remove from the heat. If you wish, you may add a couple of drops of essential oil, such as peppermint or spearmint, or a small amount of brandy to help preserve the syrup and to aid as a relaxant in cough formulas.

Step 6. Bottle the syrup and store in the refrigerator, where it will keep for several weeks, even months.

HERBAL BATHS

MOST CHILDREN LOVE BATHING and will spend hours playing in a tub of water if allowed to. As well as being fun and delightful, herbal baths can be helpful for any number of conditions, depending on the herbs that are used in the bathwater. Chamomile and lavender baths, for example, can work wonders on anxious children, soothing and calming them — and parents, too. When a child has respiratory congestion from a cold, a warm herbal bath of eucalyptus and/or thyme helps clear the congestion.

Imagine an herbal bath as a giant cup of herbal tea and you're infusing your child — or yourself — in the warm wonders of it all. Though we don't normally think of it as such, our skin is our largest organ of assimilation and elimination. When we bathe, the warm water opens our pores, and the nutrients of water and herb flow into us. Warm water is also relaxing and calming, so the very nature of bathing calms and nourishes.

To make an herbal bath, prepare a quart of strong herbal tea (see the directions on page 95), using two to three times the amount of herb you would normally use, and add the liquid to the bathwater. Alternatively, you can place the herbs in a muslin bag (or a cotton or nylon sock) and tie it to the nozzle of the tub. Run very hot water through the herbal bag until the tub is half filled, and then adjust the temperature with cold water. Have your child soak in the bath for at least 30 minutes to enjoy the full benefits of the herbs.

HERBAL PILLS

HERBAL PILLS ARE SIMPLE, practical, and easy to make. You can formulate your own blends and make them taste good enough so that even children will eat them. They are excellent for sore throats because you can formulate them with herbs that fight the infection, but still make them tasty enough to suck on and soothe the throat.

HOW TO MAKE HERBAL PILLS

Step 1. Place powdered herbs in a bowl and moisten with enough water and honey or maple syrup to make a sticky paste.

Step 2. Add a tiny drop of essential oil, such as peppermint or wintergreen, if desired, and mix well.

Step 3. Thicken with carob powder, adding enough to form a smooth paste. Knead until the mixture is smooth, like the texture of bread dough.

Step 4. Roll into small balls the size of pills. (To give each the recommended dosage, divide the amount of herbs you've used by the dosage, and roll that number of pills. For example, if you've used 10 teaspoons of herbs, and the dosage is ½ teaspoon, you'd roll 20 pills.) You can roll them in carob powder for a finished look if you like.

Step 5. Place the pills on a baking tray and set to dry in the oven at very low heat (even the pilot light will work) or even just in the sun. These pills, once dried, will store indefinitely in the refrigerator.

TINCTURES

TINCTURES ARE CONCENTRATED EXTRACTS of herbs that are simple to make and easy to take, and they have a long shelf life. People with busy lives find it easier to take an herbal tincture than a tea — you simply dilute the desired dosage of the tincture in a small amount of warm water, tea, or juice and drink it.

Most tinctures are made with alcohol as the primary solvent, or menstruum. Alcohol is a strong solvent and extracts most of the important chemical constituents in plants. If for whatever reason you don't want to give your child an alcohol-based tincture, effective tinctures can also be made with vegetable glycerin or apple cider vinegar as the solvent. They are not as strong as alcohol-based preparations, but they do work. You can also combine solvents; for instance, you can make a tincture using equal parts alcohol and vegetable glycerin; you'll have the strong action of the alcohol combined with the sweet, soothing effects of the glycerin.

HOW TO MAKE GLYCERIN-BASED TINCTURES

Some people feel that glycerites (glycerin-based tinctures) are better suited for children. When properly made, they're quite strong enough. Because of the sweet nature of glycerin, they taste far better than alcohol tinctures. And they have a fairly stable shelf life. My dear friend Sunny Mavor developed an excellent line of herbal tinctures just for children and made them all with a glycerin base. Her product line, Herbs for Kids, has become quite popular and can be found in most natural health food stores.

Several methods can be used to make tinctures. Though I have run several companies and can make exacting standardized tinctures, weighing and measuring each ingredient, using fancy equipment, and keeping meticulous records, when I am in my kitchen, making my own home remedies, I use the traditional or simpler's method. It makes as fine a tincture as any made in a lab and it's so much easier and fun. All that is required to make a tincture in the simpler's method is the herbs, the solvent (menstruum), and a jar with a tight-fitting lid.

Step 1. Chop your herbs finely. I recommend using fresh herbs whenever possible. High-quality dried herbs will work well also, but one of the advantages of tincturing is the ability to preserve the fresh attributes of the plant. If you are using fresh herbs with a very high moisture content, such as comfrey or marsh mallow, you may wish to leave them out in a warm spot to wilt for a couple of hours first, to let some of that moisture evaporate. Then place the chopped herbs in a clean, dry jar.

Step 2. If you're using alcohol as your menstruum, select one that is 80 to 100 proof, such as vodka, gin, or brandy. If you're using vegetable glycerin, dilute it with water before pouring it over the herbs, in a ratio of about 2 parts glycerin to 1 part water. If you're using vinegar, warm it

(continued on next page)

first to facilitate the release of herbal constituent.

Pour in enough of the menstruum to cover the herbs by 2 to 3 inches. They should be completely submerged. (If the herbs float to the top, let them settle for a day or two, and then add more menstruum if needed.) Cover the jar with a tight-fitting lid.

Step 3. Place the jar in a warm place and let the herbs and liquid soak (macerate) for 4 to 6 weeks — the longer, the better. Shake daily. It's probably not essential to shake them daily, but I like the idea of infusing my medicine with healing thoughts, and while shaking them I am usually offering prayers for good medicine. On a practical note, shaking allows the solvent to mix thoroughly with the herbs and prevents them settling on the bottom of the jar.

Step 4. Strain the herbs from the solvent by pouring the mixture through a large stainless-steel strainer lined with cheesecloth or muslin. Reserve the liquid, which is now a potent tincture, and compost the herbs. Rebottle and be sure to label or you'll quickly forget what's in that jar! Include the name of the herb, the solvent used, and the date. Store in a cool, dark location, where the tincture will keep for a year or more.

Because of their concentration, follow the dosage guidelines on pages 91–93 carefully when administering tinctures. Remember to always dilute them in warm water, tea, or juice when giving them to children. They are too strong to use straight out of the bottle with children.

HERBAL ENEMAS

AT ONE TIME, EVERY PARENT KNEW how to administer an enema to a child to bring down a fever, help fight infection, or quickly hydrate a dehydrated child. But today enemas, like so many other useful and helpful home practices, have fallen by the wayside, and parents more often than not rely on pharmaceuticals for their children's health. Nevertheless, enemas are a very effective way to administer the healing essences of herbs — and fluids — into a sick and feverish body. A catnip enema, for example, remains one of the best and most effective ways to bring down a child's fever.

With enemas, experience is helpful. If you've never before given an enema to a child, consult with your pediatrician or health care provider for instructions. An enema should not be given to a child under three years of age unless recommended by your health care practitioner. *Please note:* Enemas are not recommended for constipation.

HOW TO PREPARE AN HERBAL ENEMA

Step 1. Combine catnip leaf with water, using 3 tablespoons of herb per pint of water, and heat very slowly over low heat for 15 minutes. Remove from the heat and let cool to room temperature. Strain.

Step 2. Pour less than 1 cup of the catnip infusion into an enema bag. Prepare your child; you'll want to have him or her lie on towels or, even better, get in the tub.

Step 3. Place the enema bag at shoulder height so that the liquid can flow smoothly. Lubricate the tip with an herbal salve or oil and insert into the child's rectum. This is generally not painful or even uncomfortable for the child. *Slowly* release a gentle flow of liquid. The primary thing to be aware of is to not let the liquid flow quickly or forcefully; keep it at a slow, steady stream.

Step 4. The longer your child holds in the liquid, the better. But even if the child holds the liquid in for just a couple of minutes, the medicine will be effective. So after withdrawing the tip of the enema bag, fold a towel and press firmly over the child's anus for a few minutes to aid in retention.

INFUSED OILS

HERBAL OILS ARE MADE by infusing herbs in oil. It's that simple. And once you've made herbal oil, you're a step away from making salves and ointments.

Many people prefer to make oils using fresh herbs, and you certainly can. But I find that in most cases high-quality dried herbs, which are more concentrated and don't contain water that could spoil the salve, make a better oil and/or salve. I do enjoy making herbal oils from fresh herbs, going outside and collecting fresh plantain and yarrow, comfrey, and chickweed, but I usually will dry-wilt these herbs before adding them to the oil. Dry wilting allows some of the moisture to evaporate, so there's less chance of spoilage due to the water content of fresh herbs.

HOW TO MAKE INFUSED OILS

DOUBLE BOILER METHOD

This is the classic method of preparing an infused oil.

Step 1. Chop the herbs and put them in the top part of a double boiler. A double boiler is strongly recommended over a regular pan because the oil can overheat quickly, destroying the herbs and oil. You don't want deep-fried herbs or burned oil, and believe me, it happens very quickly unless you're using a double boiler.

Step 2. Cover the herbs with an inch or two of high-quality cooking oil (I prefer olive oil).

(continued on next page)

Step 3. Slowly heat the oil to a low simmer, with just a few bubbles. Keeping the heat low, gently simmer for 30 minutes to 1 hour, checking frequently to be sure the oil is not overheating. When the oil looks and smells "herby" — it will become deep green or golden and smell strongly of herbs — then you know the herbal properties have been transferred to the oil. The lower the heat, the longer the infusion, and the better the oil.

Step 4. Remove the oil from the heat and let cool.

Step 5. Strain the herbs from the oil, using a large stainless-steel strainer lined with cheesecloth. Discard the spent herbs and bottle your herbal oil.

Watch for Condensation

Occasionally, in a moist climate like New England, where I live, condensation will gather on the inside top of the jar as the oil infuses. Since water can introduce bacteria to the oil, if you see this happen, open the jar and use a clean dry cloth to wipe up any water. Alternatively, some people prefer to use thick layers of cheesecloth as the covering rather than a tight-fitting lid, so any condensation can evaporate. But this happens only occasionally, and only in a moist climate.

SOLAR INFUSION METHOD

This, I must admit, is my favorite method for making herbal oils. I learned how to make oils this way from one of my earliest teachers, Juliette de Bairacli Levy. She would place her jars of infusing oils in sandboxes to concentrate the heat, a technique used in her native Greece and the rest of the Mediterranean. In this solar extraction method, you use the great luminary energy of the sun to extract the herb's properties into the oil. There must be something healing about that.

Step 1. Place the herbs in a widemouthed glass jar and add enough high-quality cooking oil (I prefer olive oil) to cover the herbs by 1 to 2 inches. Cover tightly.

Step 2. Place the jar in a warm, sunny spot and let steep for 2 weeks. (For a super double-strength infusion, at the end of 2 weeks strain out the herbs, add a fresh batch of herbs, and infuse for 2 more weeks. This will give you very potent medicinal oil.)

Step 3. Strain the herbs from the oil, using a large stainless-steel strainer lined with cheesecloth. Discard the spent herbs and bottle your herbal oil.

Because oils generally go rancid quite quickly when exposed to heat and light, you would expect these solar-infused oils to spoil within a couple of weeks. However, so long as the herb is infusing in the oil, they don't go rancid. Once poured and strained, they are as susceptible to rancidity as any oil, but during the actual process of maceration they remain stable. I've never met anyone who can explain this phenomenon to me, so I have to assume it's something to do with the antioxidant properties of the herbs.

Storing Herbal Oils

In general, oils tend to spoil quickly and don't have a long shelf life (with the exception of olive and coconut, which are remarkably stable). Most oils, if exposed to heat and light, will begin to go rancid within a few weeks; unfortunately, many are already rancid when they're purchased. Rancid oils are a major cause of free radical damage in the body and related health issues. All oils should be stored in a cool, dark place to prolong their shelf life. Refrigeration is best, but in most kitchens real estate in the "ice box" is in high demand. So find a place that's cool and dark to store those precious oils. If stored properly in a cool, dark space, herbal oils will keep for several months.

SALVES AND OINTMENTS

ONCE YOU'VE MADE HERBAL OIL, you're a step away from a salve. Salves, or ointments (two words for the same thing), are made of beeswax, herbs, and vegetable oil. The oil is used as the solvent, extracting the medicinal properties of the herbs, and also provides a healing, emollient base. The beeswax adds a soothing and protective quality and the firmness necessary to form the salve.

HOW TO MAKE SALVES AND OINTMENTS

Step 1. Begin by making an infused herbal oil, following the instructions starting on page 111.

Step 2. For each cup of herbal oil, add ¼ cup beeswax. Heat the oil and beeswax together over very low heat until the beeswax has melted. Stir together.

Step 3. Thanks to the beeswax, the mixture will thicken as it cools. To check that it's going to have the right consistency, do a quick test: Place 1 tablespoon of the mixture in the freezer for just a minute or two. Then test it. If it seems too soft, add more beeswax, reheating as necessary until the beeswax melts. If it seems too hard, add more oil.

Step 4. Once you're satisfied with the results of your consistency test, remove from the heat and pour into small glass jars or tins. Obviously, you're working with very hot oil, so be careful.

Step 5. Let cool, and store in a cool, dark place. Stored properly, salves will keep for several months.

How Much Is a Drop?

Have you ever been frustrated when a recipe provides only one type of measurement? Here are some basic conversions to keep in mind:

TEASPOONS	DROPPERSFUL	MILLILITERS
¼	1 (35 drops)	1
½	2.5 (88 drops)	2.5
1	5 (175 drops)	5

(Who was it that counted those drops? I'd like to thank her!)

Converting Recipe Measurements to Metric

Use the following formulas for converting US measurements to metric. Since the conversions are not exact, it's important to convert the measurements for all of the ingredients to maintain the same proportions as the original recipe.

WHEN THE MEASUREMENT GIVEN IS	TO CONVERT IT TO	MULTIPLY IT BY
teaspoons	milliliters	4.93
tablespoons	milliliters	14.79
cups	milliliters	236.59
	liters	0.236
pints	milliliters	473.18
	liters	0.473
quarts	milliliters	946.36
	liters	0.946
ounces	grams	28.35
inches	centimeters	2.54

RECOMMENDED READING

Bove, Mary. *An Encyclopedia of Natural Healing for Children and Infants.* Keats Publishing, 1996.

Clark, Demetria. *Herbal Healing for Children.* Healthy Living Publications, 2011.

Combs, Dawn. *Conceiving Healthy Babies.* New Society Publishers, 2014.

De Bairacli Levy, Juliette. *Nature's Children.* Ash Tree Publishing, 1997.

Dodt, Colleen. *Natural BabyCare.* Storey Publishing, 1997.

Gladstar, Rosemary. *Rosemary Gladstar's Herbal Recipes for Vibrant Health.* Storey Publishing, 2008.

———. *Rosemary Gladstar's Medicinal Herbs: A Beginner's Guide.* Storey Publishing, 2012.

Hartung, Tammi. *Homegrown Herbs.* Storey Publishing, 2011.

Mazzarella, Barbara. *Bach Flower Remedies for Children.* Healing Arts Press, 1994.

McIntyre, Anne. *The Herbal for Mother and Child.* Element Press, 1992.

Romm, Aviva Jill. *Naturally Healthy Babies and Children.* Celestial Arts, 2003.

Tierra, Lesley. *A Kid's Herb Book for Children of All Ages.* Robert D. Reed Publishers, 2000.

White, Linda, and Sunny Mavor. *Kids, Herbs, Health.* Interweave Press, 1999.

Zand, Janet, Rachel Walton, and Robert Roundtree. *Smart Medicine for a Healthier Child.* Avery Publishing Group, 1994.

RESOURCES

WHERE TO BUY HERBS

I generally suggest purchasing herbal products from local sources, as it helps support bioregional herbalism and community-based herbalists. However, if you need to search further afield, here are some of my favorite sources for high-quality herbs and herbal products.

Avena Botanicals
207-594-0694
www.avenabotanicals.com

Healing Spirits Herb Farm and Education Center
607-566-2701
www.healingspiritsherbfarm.com

Herbalist and Alchemist
908-689-9020
www.herbalist-alchemist.com

Herb Pharm
800-348-4372
www.herb-pharm.com

Jean's Greens Herbal Tea Works & Herbal Essentials
518-479-0471
www.jeansgreens.com

Mountain Rose Herbs
800-879-3337
www.mountainroseherbs.com

Pacific Botanicals
541-479-7777
www.pacificbotanicals.com

Woodland Essence
315-845-1515
www.woodlandessence.com

Zack Woods Herb Farm
802-851-7536
www.zackwoodsherbs.com

EDUCATIONAL RESOURCES

American Herb Association
www.ahaherb.com

American Herbalists Guild
617-520-4372
www.americanherbalistsguild.com
The only national organization for professional, peer-reviewed herbal practitioners; offers a directory of members

California School of Herbal Studies
707-887-7457
www.cshs.com
One of the oldest herb schools in the United States, founded by Rosemary Gladstar in 1978

Herb Research Foundation
www.herbs.org/herbnews
A clearinghouse of herb information; publishes an excellent newsletter

Sage Mountain Retreat Center & Botanical Sanctuary
802-479-9825
www.sagemountain.com
Apprenticeships and classes with Rosemary Gladstar and other well-known herbalists, as well as a home-study course

United Plant Savers
740-742-3455
www.unitedplantsavers.org
A nonprofit organization dedicated to the conservation and cultivation of endangered North American medicinal plants. Provides conferences, journals, and other educational services to members.

INDEX

Page numbers in *italic* indicate illustrations; page numbers in **bold** indicate charts.

A

acidophilus supplement, 41, 49,
    54, 56, 62
All-Purpose Healing Salve, 52–53
allergies, 5, 33, 60, 93, 95
    herbs that help, 23, 26
    the patch test, 7
allopathic medicine, 3–4, 6
aloe for burns, 80–81
American Association of Poison
    Control Centers (AAPCC), 6
anise, 11, 41, 43, 96
antiviral herbs, 16, 20–21, 32
apple cider vinegar, 62, 67, 106
arrowroot, 49–50
astragalus, 11–12, 68, 76

B

Baby's Bath Herbs, 85
Baby's Blessed Bath & Bottom
    Oil, 87
Baby's Sweet Sleep Pillow, 86
baths, herbal, 103–4
blackberry root, 54–55
burdock root, 76, 79
    herbal formulas, 46, 68, 70
burns, 5, 79–80
    All-Purpose Healing Salve, 52
    Healing Clay, 81
    herbs that help, 22, 29

C

calcium-rich tea, 36–37
calendula, *86*
    herbal formulas, 52, 69, 71,
        84–87
Calming Tonic Tea, 82–83
candy balls, how to make, 98–101
catnip, 12, 38, 41
    catnip tea, 36

herbal enemas, 109–10
herbal formulas, 43, 67,
    82–83
chamomile, 8, *9*, 12–13
    baths, 44, 103
    combined with other herbs,
        15, 20, 36, 38–39
    herbal formulas, 43, 47, 52,
        82–83, 85–87
chicken pox, 4, 68–71
cinnamon,
    herbal formulas, 28–29, 37,
        42, 55, 59, 75, 78, 83, 96
colds and flus, 72–78
    Cough Be Gone & Sore Throat
        Syrup, 75
    lung and chest congestion,
        77–78
    runny nose and sinus conges-
        tion, 77
colic, 39–45
    herbs that help, 11–14, 18, 41
    Hyland's homeopathic colic
        tablets, 38, 44
    Marsh Mallow Gruel, 42
    old-fashioned techniques,
        44–45
    Seed Tea, 43
coltsfoot, 84, *84*
comfrey, *51*, 107, 111
    herbal formulas, 50–52, 71,
        81, 87
constipation, 56–59
    suggested treatment options,
        57–58
    Tea to Relieve Constipation, 59
Cough Be Gone & Sore Throat
    Syrup, 75
Cowling's Rules of dosage

amounts, 91
cradle cap, 45–47
    Cradle Cap Oil, 47
    Tea for Cradle Cap, 46
cuts and scrapes, 79–81

D

decoctions, 97
diaper rash, 48–53
    All-Purpose Healing Salve,
        52–53
    Baby Powder, 50–51
    common irritants, 48–49
    herbal powders, 49–51
diarrhea, 53–55
    Blackberry Root Tincture, 54
    Diarrhea Remedy Tea, 55
dill, 14, 41, 43
Disinfectant Powder, 71
dosages
    chart for adults, 93, **93**
    dangers of concentrated
        doses, 8
    determining a child's dosage,
        91–92, **92**

E

earaches and infection, 60–65
    causes of, 62–63
    Ear Infection Formula, 85
    Garlic and Mullein Flower
        Oil, 84
    herbal formulas, 64–65, 84
    when to seek medical atten-
        tion, 4–5
echinacea, 14–15, *15*
    combined with other herbs, 11,
        16–17, 51
    herbal formulas, 51, 65,
        67–70, 73–75, 78